PSYCHOSOMATIC YOGA

A practical handbook of specific Yoga techniques for improving mind-body relationship, maintaining psychological equilibrium, training the concentrative faculties, and exploring the possible release of latent nervous energy within the body.

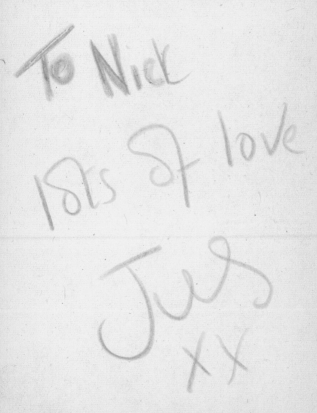

To Nick

lots of love

Jess

xx

PSYCHOSOMATIC YOGA

A Guide to Eastern Path Techniques

By

JONN MUMFORD
(Swami Anandakapila Saraswati)

SAMUEL WEISER INC.
740 Broadway, New York, N.Y. 10003

First published 1974
This Edition, completely revised,
enlarged and reset, 1979

ISBN 0 85030 208 0 (UK)
ISBN 0 87728 459 8 (USA)

Photoset by
Specialised Offset Services Limited, Liverpool
and printed in Great Britain by
Weatherby Woolnough, Wellingborough
Northamptonshire

CONTENTS

Dedicated to
Swami Satyananda Saraswati
of Bihar Yoga School
Monghyr

INTRODUCTION

It need hardly be said that Yoga is a vast and intricate subject which encompasses life in general and man's relationship with life in particular.

Yoga means 'Union'. It is derived from the classical Sanskrit root *Yuji*, which still survives in our Latin as *Jungere* and in the English word 'Yoke' (i.e., an instrument which links or unites). 'Yoga' is just an instrument.

Yoga is union with what? It is union with life in its entirety. Man represents the most highly evolved of life's earthbound creations. As such, his attempts to integrate himself (and in so doing become at one with the vortex of life from whence he sprang) have varied in aspect from century to century, environment to environment, and civilization to civilization.

Thousands of years ago this problem of shifting emphasis, depending upon circumstantial need, was recognized by the sages of Yoga, each suited to particular individuals and their needs. *Hatha, Bhakti, Karma, Gnana, Raja* and *Laya* are but a few of the many aspects of Yoga which will be familiar to the student who has had some previous acquaintance with the subject.

Broadly speaking, we may say that man's problems in previous periods of history have consisted in overcoming and conquering physical obstacles such as his ever unpredictable environment and his even less predictable neighbours.

Within the last century a new era has dawned. Man is slowly but surely overcoming all physical obstacles, but is now coming up against the unconquered realms of his own mind.

Psychiatry has calculated that sixty to seventy per cent of today's diseases are of mental origin, and this is only the most conservative estimate.

Psychology suggests that five out of twelve people need professional help in the form of psychological counselling or psychiatric treatment. One out of twelve will spend some time in a mental hospital.

Switzerland and the United States have the highest standard of living in the world and also the highest suicide rates.

What are we to infer from the above factual statements? They are sad proof that man's problems for the new age are not physical but mental. I once heard a very clever lecturer remark that 'whereas it used to be the problems of man it is now Man the problem'. It is with this thought in mind that I have written this book and entitled it 'PSYCHOSOMATIC YOGA'.

Reference to a dictionary will enlighten the reader regarding the Greek roots of the word 'psychosomatic', and reveal that this word embodies the entire concept of mind-body relationship. The sum-total implication of 'psychosomatic' is that there exists a curious co-relation between the emotions and the physiological functions of the body, which makes Newton's 'For every action there is an equal and opposite reaction' an axiom of psychology rather than physics.

This text has been written as a practical handbook for those who are desirous of obtaining information on the specific use of Yoga techniques for the maintenance of psychological equilibrium, training of the concentrative faculties, and exploration of the possible release of latent nervous energy within the body.

Several of the techniques have never, to my knowledge, been printed before, and certainly detailed instructions concerning these methods have hitherto seldom been revealed, as they are considered esoteric and hence transmitted from *guru* to *chela* as an oral teaching.

I feel that I have not, strictly speaking, written with the beginner in mind, but rather for those who have traversed the 'Path' at least a little. Understanding this, the student who is completely new to the subject should avail himself of the many excellent books by internationally known authors such as Shri Yogendra, Shri Vivekananda, Dr Paul Brunton and Dr Theos Bernard.

Lastly it is my hope that students of the Western occult tradition may find these notes a convenient reference and guide to the most practical and effective techniques of the Eastern path. It is my conjecture that these techniques would be useful for experimentation and assimilation among Western occultists. This is not unreasonable when we consider that our Western occult heritage is about equally in debt to Dravidian-Aryan sources as it is to Egyptian and Semitic culture.

JONN MUMFORD
Hardwar, Uttar Pradesh State,
India

CHAPTER ONE

SUKHASANA

Hatha is perhaps the best known aspect of Yoga among Westerners. To most students it is simply a difficult system of physical control involving the use of static poses (*asanas*) and the learning of specialized breathing techniques (*pranayama*).

Few realize that the base upon which *Hatha Yoga* rests is an axiom stating that if the mind can influence the body (as admitted by psychiatrists) then the converse is equally true. The body influences the mind.

If we are nervous, depressed, or suffer from anxiety, our mental state is reflected in the function, control and appearance of our physical being. At a later stage (in chronic anxiety for instance) our habituated mental state may produce organic changes in the body resulting in such disablements as stomach ulcers, colitis, heart disease and perhaps even cancer.

Hatha Yoga re-establishes the mental stability of the individual and thus reverses the process which results in psychosomatic disease. This is accomplished by first teaching the student to acquire control of his body. Control of the body, in turn, requires effort at controlling the mind, since no muscle is flexed, no nerve activated, or blood circulated unless under the control (voluntary or involuntary) of the mind.

The Sanskrit roots of *Hatha* break down into *Ha* and *Tha*. *Ha* refers to the sun, a positive masculine symbol, while *Tha* refers to the moon, a negative feminine symbol. Generally *Hatha* is understood as indicating the union of the positive, sundrenched inbreath (*Ha*) with the negative outbreath (*Tha*). Given a deeper interpretation we see that *Ha* esoterically symbolizes the positive mind uniting with its negative vehicle *Tha*, the body. Herein lies the clue to the true esoteric teaching of Adam (the mind) and Eve (the body) as depicted in Genesis.

Hatha Yoga may be defined as the science of uniting and co-ordinating the physical and mental aspects of man's being through consciously attempted discipline of the body.

It was during this century that the Russian scientist, Pavlov, rediscovered the principle of 'conditioning' and the 'conditioned reflex' known for several thousand years by the *Hatha Yogins*. It is upon this fact of being able to condition the body and consequently the mind, that we begin our study of the first exercise, *Sukhasana*.

The 'Easy Pose'
Sukhasana literally means 'Easy Pose' (*Sukha* – Easy; *Asana* – Pose). It is one of a number of meditative poses. Like all meditative poses it shares certain common characteristics.

Specific Advantages
1. A solid, triangular base for trunk and head.
2. The spine is kept straight and thus nerve flow along spine and between vertebrae is uninhibited.
3. The lungs are free for exercises in deep breathing as taught in *pranayama*.
4. Said to aid awakening of *kundalini* (latent nervous energy locked within Central Nervous System).

Sukhasana has specific physiological and psychological advantages. Physiologically the internal viscera are relaxed because of the 'tailor-fashion' crossed legs, while psychologically the mind and body are brought into a harmonious state of stability through the consciously willed attempt to remain motionless.

Sukhasana is the ideal technique for those who wish to condition themselves for shutting the door upon everyday business worries, and thus prepare themselves for the meditative peace to be found within the recesses of their own mind. This technique is also valuable for nervous disorders involving poor neuro-muscular co-ordination, twitches, nervous movements and 'tics'.

Technique

1. Place folded blanket on floor. Sit upon blanket with legs stretched out in front of you.
2. Bend the right leg under the left thigh and the left leg under the right thigh, thus assuming the cross-legged 'tailor pose'. Check that the knee-caps are roughly level with each other. If they are not the trunk will lean slightly to the lower side, thus disturbing body symmetry and balance.
3. Keep the spine erect and the head nicely poised upon the shoulders.
4. Place the hands, palm down, upon the knees in such a fashion that they will not slip off. Be certain that the elbows relax naturally against the body.
5. Firmly close the eyes as if you were drawing down shutters and continue to keep the eyelids under control for the duration of the session.
6. You are now introverted within yourself. Concentrate the mind upon the natural rhythm of your breath, control yourself from dreaming, reasoning or otherwise becoming mentally active, and keep the body erect, motionless and as relaxed as possible. Concentrate upon just 'being'. If you find the mind wandering and attention upon the body position and breathing insufficient for concentration, try visualizing and holding a simple

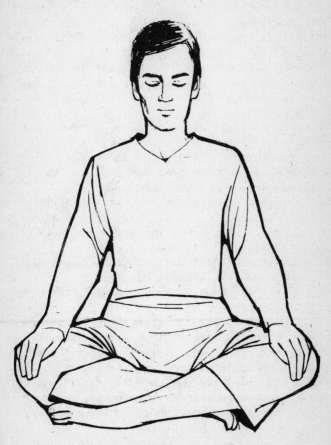

Sukhasana

object in the mind's eye, namely, a geometrical pattern, a flower, colour or image.

Minimum performance: five minutes.

Check Points

1. After commencement of exercise check elbows to see that they are relaxed and swing freely.

2. Check eyelids to see that they are steady and controlled. Any flickering of the lashes indicates mental agitation and lack of absorption in the exercise.

3. Make certain that you do not unconsciously slip into a slouch and thus bend the spine.

As with any of the classical *Hatha Asanas*, very distinct performance problems arise. Let us list them along with appropriate remedies.

1. Pressure of floor upon feet may cause pain and thus distract attention. This is overcome by practice in which the feet are gradually conditioned.

2. The spine may tend to slouch. The remedy lies in sustained, disciplined effort.

3. The mind becomes agitated and refuses to quieten. We follow the same principle of quieting a bored or upset child. We provide something suitable in the way of distraction, such as concentration upon simple objects, etc. This particular problem is the crux of the exercise. What happens is that you eventually train yourself to relax mentally upon beginning the exercise, and this conditioning becomes stronger with repetition.

Sukhasana should be practised consistently for a week before starting practice of the next exercise. All routines should be commenced with Sukhasana and the minimum time of five minutes lengthened to ten minutes maximum.

In review, remember that Sukhasana, practised in the described manner, is a specific therapy for nervous disorders arising from lack of neuro-muscular control. In this exercise control over the body is increased and willpower is strengthened. Above all the mind is trained into a quiet state of mental 'set', and this conditioning prepares the student for advanced exercises.

Traditionally admission to certain Eastern occult schools depended upon the *chela's* ability to remain motionless for a three-hour test period. The average individual, in our tension-fraught age, cannot remain mentally absorbed and physically motionless for three minutes (not to suggest three hours) or even ten minutes, as you are expected to accomplish through *Sukhasana*.

CHAPTER TWO

SAVASANA

Unfortunate as it may be, you and I are immersed in a tension-filled world. It is this very tension that forms the basis for psychosomatic disturbances. We are left asking ourselves what we can do about our individual tensions and what we may do about world tension, which, after all, is only the result of accumulated individual tension. Psychiatry offers tranquillizers but *Hatha Yoga* offers drugless, inner relaxation through the thousands-of-years-old process known as *Savasana*.

Seldom do you find physical tension apart from mental tension and curiously enough mental tension always arises first and is the cause of physical tension. *Savasana*, like *Sukhasana*, reverses the usual mind-body arc and teaches the individual to gain conscious control over the vital zones of his body and thus relax the mind into *Yoga-Nidra* (sleep of the Yogis) through first relaxing the physical body.

This again confirms our elementary Hatha principle that the mind and the body are linked and whatever happens to one will affect the other as surely as goading one of two yoked oxen will force the other to move along with it. Knowing this we may confidently proceed to use *Savasana* as a specific panacea for such psychosomatic ailments as neurasthenia, hypertension, insomnia, and high blood-pressure.

Savasana means 'Corpse Pose' (*Sava* – Corpse;

Asana – Pose) and it has also been called *Mritasana* or 'Dead Pose' (*Mrit* – Dead).

The student will discover that the classical names given to this exercise rather dramatically emphasize the relaxation accruing from its practice.

Specific Advantages

1. A deep state of muscular relaxation is brought about.
2. The blood-pressure is lowered (individuals with unusually low blood-pressure may suffer discomfort from practice of *Savasana*) while at the same time heart-beat and respiration are considerably slowed.
3. A transfer of *prana* (nervous energy) to the internal organs takes place.
4. The nervous system is rested and rejuvenated.
5. The mind is brought to the point of complete relaxation from which it may go into a deep, dreamless sleep. (This is optional, depending on the student's desire.)

The practice of *Savasana* is most conveniently divided into two steps or stages.

Elementary Technique

At this stage you learn to relax the body as a unit and give in completely to the force of gravity. If you observe a cat or a baby sleeping you will see that upon awakening they leave a deep impression in the cushion or mat slept upon. Animals and babies instinctively let go completely and allow gravity to do the work.

Technique One

1. Lie supine (face up) on the floor upon a suitable folded blanket. Loose clothing should be worn and the room temperature ought to be comfortably warm.
2. Place your feet about twenty inches apart and allow the ankles and toes to relax to the outside.

3. Place the hands, palm up, about ten inches out from the body on either side.

4. Check that the shoulders are flat and the small of the back relaxed into the floor.

5. Adjust the head to a comfortable position.

6. Completely surrender your body weight to the floor.

7. Commence concentrating upon your upper and lower extremities (namely, the arms and legs) and with each exhalation (normal expiration) feel your arms and legs becoming heavier and heavier. Imagine yourself sinking into the floor.

It should be noted that the placing of the extremities permits the individual to take maximum advantage of the natural pull of gravity. *Hatha Yoga* teaches, as a fundamental tenet, the use of natural forces such as gravity.

This exercise should be practised for a minimum of ten to fifteen minutes and should be performed for a week before starting the second phase of *Savasana*.

Advanced Technique

In the advanced step we learn to localize each part of the body and systematically relax and inhibit afferent and efferent (sensory and motor) nervous impulses. This is accomplished through commencing concentration at the feet and slowly working up to the head.

The Yogins (whose knowledge of neuro-anatomy was gained by introspection) long ago discovered the secret nerve zones of the human body and divided them into sixteen major areas called *Marmasthanani*. These positions are as follows:

(1) Feet, (2) Shins, (3) Knee-caps, (4) Thighs, (5) Abdomen, (6) Solar Plexus, (7) Upper Chest, (8) Spine, (9) Hands, (10) Forearms, (11) Upper Arms, (12) Throat, (13) Back of Head, (14) Jaw, (15) Eyes, (16) Scalp or *Bramapura*.

Technique Two

1. Repeat steps one to five as in 'Technique One'.
2. Begin with the first *Marmasthanani*, the feet, and:
(a) Create a mental picture of your toes and ankles.
(b) Increase your self-consciousness or self-awareness of the area by concentrating upon feeling internally the bone, muscle, sinew and blood.
(c) Having increased your awareness of the area, mentally will a state of relaxation, heaviness and sinking into that particular spot.
3. Switch your attention to the next zone and repeat parts a, b, and c of step two. Work your way up over the whole body in this fashion.

Allow at least half a minute for each zone and go over the body repeatedly until you relax so completely that you fall into *Yoga Nidra*.

Savasana is the ancient and natural contribution of Yoga to this very modern problem of tension and insomnia. Because of the effect *Savasana* has in slowing the metabolic processes, while at the same time conserving nervous energy, it is one of the hidden keys to the many medically authenticated cases of hibernation involving the burying alive of Yogins for weeks at a time.

A mastery of *Savasana* will enable the student to gain conscious control over his muscular and nervous system. A good test of mastery of this technique is the ability to sleep within three minutes.

CHAPTER THREE

YONI MUDRA

The eternal, age-old path of Yoga has designed techniques which permit a man not just to escape the illusion (*maya*) we term 'Life', but to escape within himself to a true inner reality wherein may be found the flaming lamp of transcendental consciousness. As man uses Yoga to probe deeper within the grottoes of his own mind he approaches closer and closer to the core of his own being until he experiences self-reintegration physically, mentally and emotionally.

One such technique of turning within is *Yoni Mudra*. *Yoni* means womb or source. This reference is to the Absolute or Brahman as the source of all existence. The word *mudra*, in this case, denotes a physical practice which has effect on the mind. *Yoni Mudra* has also been called *Sanmukhi* (*san* means six and *mukhi* means orifice or mouth) indicating that the six body orifices are closed, namely, eyes, ears, nose, mouth, anus and genital opening. Another classical name is *Parang Mukhi*. *Parang* suggests a turning away from the outside world and a closing off of the senses result in *Pratyahara* (sense withdrawal).

Specific Advantages
1. The five senses are shut off mechanically and this leads to a semi-automatic state of *Pratyahara*.
2. The nervous system is rejuvenated, particularly as the eyes are shut (and they use more nervous energy than any other sense organ).

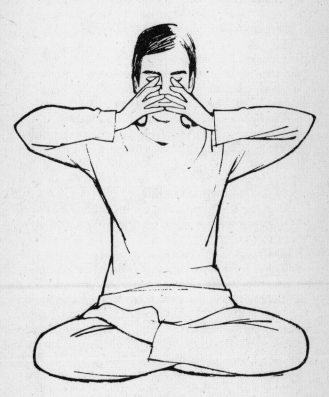

Yoni Mudra

3. Co-operation is brought about between the mind and the body as a result of the disciplined conditioning required to maintain the pose.

4. The mind is given an opportunity to introvert and experience complete cutting off from what may be a disturbing environment.

Yoni Mudra, like *Savasana*, is divided into an elementary technique and an advanced technique.

Elementary Technique

1. Sit in a meditative pose. *Padmasana* is preferred for those already experienced in *Hatha Yoga* but *Sukhasana* will be adequate for the beginner.

2. Raise the elbows level with the shoulders and at right angles with the body, jutting out on each side.

3. (a) Close the ears by inserting the thumbs in the ears.

   (b) Close the eyes with the forefingers, placing fingers along lower lids.

   (c) Place the middle fingers on either side of the bridge of the nose, leaving the nostrils open for breathing.

   (d) Press the upper lip shut with the ring fingers.

   (e) Press the lower lip shut with the little fingers.

4. Breathe slowly and evenly while concentrating the mind upon any visual images, spots or colours that may arise. If spots appear, visualize them contracting and expanding.

The pose should be held for at least five minutes and gradually worked up to fifteen minutes. You will notice that colours appear brighter after practice and a feeling of tranquillity ensues. Spend a week on the 'Elementary Stage' before attempting the 'Advanced Technique'.

Advanced Technique

1. Repeat Elementary Technique up to and including part three.

2. Commence alternate nostril breathing by

pressing shut the left nostril with the left middle finger, and inhaling slowly and evenly through the right nostril. After a full inhalation press the right nostril shut with the right middle finger, open the left nostril and exhale slowly and evenly through it. Inhale slowly and evenly through left nostril, close it, open right nostril, exhale through it and continue repeating the cycle of alternate nostril breathing.

3. After firmly establishing the breathing rhythm, begin the mental repetition of the mantra *Ham Sa*. *Ham* is mentally repeated on the inhalation and *Sa* is mentally repeated on the exhalation. The *japa* (repetition) of the mantra is to be carried on in conjunction with, and while being mindful of, the alternate nostril breathing. This particular mantra will have a deep effect upon the subconscious as well as quieting the conscious mind.

4. Absorb yourself deeper and deeper in the exercise with the object of experiencing what might be best described as a conscious moment of 'No-Thought'.

This advanced stage should be performed for fifteen minutes and a goal set of half-an-hour.

Implications of the New Steps

Let us discuss the implications of the new steps in the advanced stage.

The addition of alternate nostril breathing has a profound effect upon the body-mind relationship. As we will discuss more fully in a later section, the respiratory cycle is a major link between the physical and mental activity of humans. A man who is emotionally aroused, angry or frightened, will also breathe rapidly. Obviously any attempt at controlling the breathing will simultaneously produce a tranquillizing, balancing effect on both body and mind.

Not only does the physiological effect of a harmonized metabolism, through controlled respiration, induce relaxation, but also slow even breathing signals 'tranquillity' and 'peace' to the unconscious mind.

We may compare our mind to a monkey jumping constantly from place to place, never stopping to regenerate or concentrate its scattered energy unless a pole is placed into the ground for it to climb upon and rest.

In the early stage of *Yoni Mudra* the mind has been shut off from extraneous sensory stimulation and mental agitation farther calmed by deep, even respiration. It is now that the mind needs a 'pole' or concentrative point if it is to climb into higher states of consciousness. The 'pole' or focal point is provided in the form of mantra *Ham Sa*, which means 'He I am'. 'He' is the eternal source of all being, Brahman, the Paramatman, the Absolute. You could not have a more powerful pivot or focalizing point from which to spring into higher states of consciousness. Through this *audgita* (silent chanting) you pass from *Pratyahara* proper into *Samyama* (concentration, contemplation and meditation).

Yoni Mudra is one of the most suitable methods in *Hatha Yoga* for passing into *antaranga*, the higher branches dealt with in *Raja Yoga*. It should be mentioned that just as *Savasana* is the hidden key to yogic trance states, so *Yoni Mudra* is the key to the *siddhis* (psychic powers) of clairvoyance and clairaudience.

CHAPTER FOUR

POLARIZATION

Raja means king and thus *Raja Yoga* is the 'Kingly Yoga' or the 'Royal Way'. The 'King' or master in our lives is mind, and it is the control of mind that *Raja Yoga* teaches.

Patanjali's *Yoga Sutras* is considered the classic text on *Raja Yoga*. Its four chapters deal with the discipline of the mind and psychic potential. *Ashtanga Yoga*, as Patanjali's book is often called, is a specific study of the inner or esoteric four limbs of Yoga. These four limbs are *Pratyahara* (sometimes considered a part of *Bahira-anga* or as the transitory stage from *Hatha* to *Raja*), *Dharana* (concentration), *Dhyana* (contemplation or sustained concentration) and *Samadhi* (states of ecstasy, realization and cosmic consciousness).

Supernormal Abilities

We are going to be primarily concerned with *Dharana* or concentration. Concentration is the key to the *siddhis*, the so-called supernatural powers (really supernormal abilities latent within us all) such as photographic memory, self-anaesthesia, mental calculations, etc. According to tradition, *Raja Yoga* confers upon the student the more spectacular psychic powers in the form of telepathy, clairvoyance, psychometry and related phenomena belonging to the field of parapsychology.

Raja Yoga may be defined as the science of concentrating and focusing the conscious mind upon the unconscious mind until a mergence takes place between them, resulting in a new superconscious state of mind. As you have gathered by now, *Raja Yoga* deals exclusively with the mind and may therefore be considered as applied Eastern psychology.

In this age of Western psychologists, psychiatrists, and social workers, a few words would not be amiss concerning the essential differences between Eastern psychology, as typified by *Raja Yoga*, and contemporary Western psychology.

Modern Western psycho-analysis may be said to have really commenced with the work of Freud, some sixty years ago. The psychology of *Raja Yoga*, as expounded by Patanjali, is nearly two thousand years old and the source from which Patanjali drew his material is even older.

Western psychology is based upon theory proved empirically by tests which have provided statistical data. Eastern psychology has as its fundamental basis, personal, subjective experience. The Eastern student does not rationalize truth – he experiences it. It is an Eastern maxim that the student accepts nothing as true until he validates it by personal experience.

Differing Methodology

Western and Eastern psychology both have the goal of aiding man to solve his problems. Where they differ is in methodology.

The Western approach limits the individual to staying within his problem and understanding it through 'psycho-analysis' or the more recent, and excellent school, of 'non-directive counselling' as advocated by Carl Rogers. (This particular school is coming close to the approach of Eastern psychology.)

The Eastern approach sets no limits upon the

method of solving the problem and rather would suggest that man should transcend his personality problems through the transmutation techniques of Yoga, in general, and *Raja Yoga*, in particular.

What is needed is a synthesis of the best of Eastern and Western psychology. Where Eastern psychology lacks objective data for providing empirical proof, Western psychology lacks objective techniques which will produce subjective changes within the patient or student.

Raja Yoga, under a competent teacher, makes two claims which are emphatically denied as possible by Western psychologists. Firstly, through graded steps in visualization, the development of a photographic memory is ensured, and secondly, the raising of an individual intelligence quotient to well above average and perhaps even 'genius' level. Keeping these claims in mind the student can see just how interesting the implications of an East-West psychological synthesis would be.

Worry-absorbing Exercise

We finish our 'fifty-minute hour' with the psychiatrist and once again find ourselves alone to face the worries, frustrations, and problems of our life. What have we gained, that we personally may apply, in the way of a concrete technique for 'self-help'? *Raja Yoga* fills the very gap of Western psychology with a worry-absorbing exercise that we call 'polarization'.

Let us employ an analogy as an aid to understanding the mechanics of 'polarization'. Suppose we have a magnet and an ordinary piece of iron bar and desire to magnetize or 'polarize' the metal. You will recall enough of elementary science to know that the molecular arrangement of a magnet is in alignment, so that a single force field is produced. This is not the case with the iron bar as its molecular structure is not harmoniously patterned, and consequently the individual force fields of each molecule are working at cross purposes to each other.

If we commence, slowly and systematically, to stroke the iron bar with the magnet, we shall gradually align the bar's molecular structure and a state of polarization will result, turning the bar into a magnet.

The magnet represents our mind, while the iron bar symbolizes the emotional and psychic aspects of our physical being. *Raja Yoga* teaches 'polarization' as an exercise that brings about harmony and balance between all positive and negative aspects of the psychosomatic body-mind link. Yoga teaches that just as we may magnetize or 'polarize' the body with mental currents, this is possible through the functioning of the psychic nerves or *Nadis*.

Regardless of the theory, a short trial of the psychological rejuvenation brought about by this secret exercise will convince the student that it is one of the most valuable techniques in *Raja Yoga*.

Specific Advantages

1. Practised regularly, polarization will give relief from chronic anxiety and depression. The mind is forced to absorb itself during the exercise and thus the 'worry circle' is broken up.
2. Polarization may be practised in such a fashion as to induce *Yoga Nidra* and therefore is useful in conjunction with *Savasana* for neurasthenia and insomnia.
3. Concentration and visualization are greatly increased and at the same time internal awareness of the body is developed.
4. Yoga theory suggests that the nerves are purified (*nadisuddhi*) through direct control of the nervous energy or *prana* within the body.

Technique

1. Lie supine (face up) on the floor upon a folded blanket. The body should be so orientated that the head is north and the feet south. This is again the Yoga principle of taking advantage of natural forces – in this case the earth's magnetic field.

2. Place the feet together and the hands, palm up, close to the body (actually touching the sides).

3. If you are practising polarization for the relief of anxiety, neurasthenia or insomnia, prepare yourself by doing *Savasana* in reverse. Start with the vital zones of the head and work down to the feet, maintaining consciousness and not falling into *Yoga Nidra*.

4. Start polarization proper by visualizing on a slow, even inhalation, positive, pranic, sun energy, warm and golden yellow in colour, being drawn through the top of the head, down through the body and out of the soles of the feet.

5. On a slow, even exhalation, visualize negative, apanic, moon energy, cool and blue in colour, being drawn up through the soles of the feet, through the body and out of the top of the head.

6. Continue the respective visualizations of inhalation and exhalation and at the same time try to feel the passage of these energies sweeping the body and producing a sensation similar to an electric current.

   With the coloured inhalation feel a tingle vibrate from head to toe, and from toe to head with coloured exhalation. Synchronize the breath, visualization, and sensation of energy flow.

Reaping the Benefits

For the treatment of the aforementioned psychological symptoms, remain absorbed in the exercise until you lose consciousness and drop into the refreshing state of *Yoga Nidra*.

For improvement of concentration and

visualization keep the conscious mind focused on the visualizations and internal sensations, without permitting sleep to ensue.

Polarization should be practised fifteen minutes to half-an-hour each day for at least a week before adding new exercises.

The first indication of mastering this technique will be the intensification of concentration to the point where you feel a distinct electric current running through the body with each inhalation and exhalation. This is a sensation which must be experienced to be understood.

The commencement of our studies in *Raja Yoga* makes it possible to refine the *Hatha* technique of *Savasana*, a method of achieving physical relaxation with inevitable mental relaxation following. We are now to start distinguishing between physical tension and mental tension.

As a rule *Savasana* and polarization may be used together to ensure the attainment of *Yoga Nidra*. The stipulation is that in cases of mental tension (namely, anxiety, worry) *Savasana* must be done from the head down rather than from the feet up.

This is for the simple reason that we subconsciously and consciously associate our mental activity (and hence our mental tensions) with the head region. It is obvious that mental tension is better relaxed by carrying our conscious awareness away from the skull area and down to the feet.

CHAPTER FIVE

CONCENTRATION

Concentration is a focusing of the mind by the mind. In other words, concentration always involves an internal adjustment. Most people forget, however, that just as a delicate, high-powered microscope must be gently brought into focus, so gentleness is a prerequisite of true concentration. Yoga emphasizes *Ahimsa* or non-violence whatever the nature of the activity.

Dharana Yantra

How may we test for a relaxed state of mind ready to begin *Dharana* or concentration practice? Close your eyes and deliberately create a warm, smooth, velvety darkness as if you were looking up into a moonless, starless tropical night. The more tense your mind is, the more your inner blackness will be disturbed by colours and white spots.

It was to aid gaining the necessary relaxed state of mind that Yogis recommended meditation in dark caves, monastery cells and similar places. The creation of a pure, black field of mental vision will often so relax the mind that pain sensations from psychosomatic headaches are inhibited.

The student may be wondering what specific result was served by *Dharana* in the Yoga scheme of self-development. The mind may be thought of as a wave-covered (emotionally turbulent) lake. Such stormy waters perturb boats (the external objects perceived through the five senses) and also obscure a view of the lake bottom.

Through concentration the waters of the mind

are calmed and we achieve a clear focus upon the boats or objects of the senses. At a later stage (*Dhyana*) we focus within our own being and catch a glimpse of the pearls lying upon the lake bottom of our life.

Specific Advantages
1. Develops concentration to the level required in *Raja Yoga*.
2. Increases the ability to visualize by transferring an external image to the inner mind's eye.

Preparation
It will be necessary for the student to construct a special *Dharana Yantra* or concentration diagram (a yantra is a geometrical figure used for concentrative purposes). The *Dharana Yantra* is made by pasting a white two-inch square of paper upon the centre of a black piece of paper of average writing size.

Technique
1. Assuming a meditative pose, or sit in a chair, facing a blank, light-coloured wall at a distance of two or three feet.
2. Pin the *Dharana Yantra* diagram upon the wall in such a fashion that the centre of the white square is at eye level. Have sufficient light thrown upon the wall from behind you to see the diagram clearly.
3. Close your eyes and spend two or three minutes creating a warm, velvety blackness. Relax and gently push all disturbing or distracting images aside by repeatedly creating the black field of inner vision.
4. Open your eyes and perform *tratak* or fixation upon the centre of the diagram for three or five minutes. Gaze steadily and firmly, inhibiting the blinking reflex somewhat (but avoiding strain), until an aura forms around the edges of the white square.

5. Slowly, and without strain, transfer your gaze to a blank portion of the wall on either side and concentrate upon the after-image (a black square) which should appear on the wall. Hold your concentration for as long as the image is perceptible. When it becomes faint, use your imagination to strengthen it.

6. When the after-image has faded completely again, close your eyes and mentally recreate it. Attempt to hold it as steadily as possible on the screen of your conscious mind.

The practice of *Dharana Yantra* should be continued for at least a week before starting the technique for *Internal Dharana*. Practice time should be extended to fifteen minutes, and you should spend as much time upon each stage of the exercise as is necessary.

Internal Dharana: Specific Advantages

1. Develops concentration and visualization to the point where a photographic memory becomes a distinct possibility.

2. May be specifically used to stimulate latent memory tracts of the subconscious and thus recall forgotten material.

Technique

1. Lie down, supine, in a semi-dark room.

2. Close your eyes and with great care create a mental field of warm, velvety blackness as in step three of *Dharana Yantra*.

3. Project upon your black field a white square about the size of writing-paper and centred ten to twelve inches out from your eyes. Concentrate upon holding the image steady and preventing it from moving to either side or up and down.

4. Holding the white square, framed by the black background, imagine a black circle or black hole in the centre of the white square. The black spot

should be roughly the size of a fifty pence piece. Concentrate upon the black circle, holding the composite visualization of black background, white square and black centre.

5. End the exercise by suddenly releasing the entire visualization and watching the subconscious images that may flash across the mind's eye.

This particular form of *Internal Dharana* may be cultivated to the point where you close your eyes for a few seconds and instantly recall the desired material that had slipped beyond conscious recall.

All memories, when forgotten, have simply passed from the conscious into the subconscious storehouse. When we forget something, in an examination for instance, what has happened is that the conscious mind has frozen momentarily and thus shut off communication with the memory tracts of the brain. This exercise 'thaws out' the conscious mind by relaxing the tension and permitting a free flow along the association stream of preconscious and sub-conscious memory reservoirs.

The next time you forget a desired fact or name, close your eyes, give the sharp mental command that you 'will remember' and then absorb your mind in this particular *Internal Dharana* exercise. After completing the visualization, concentrate intensely upon holding it steady for a few seconds, and then shatter the picture and wait (with eyes still closed) for the desired association to pop itself into your conscious mind. With practice, recollection will take place in ten to fifteen seconds.

The S.C.M. Principle

The ability to create intense mental images is half the key to memory power. This ability is easy once you understand the fundamental mechanics of visualization.

'S.C.M.' stands for 'Size, Colour, Motion' – the

three requirements for successful mental imaging. If we are to leave an impression upon our memory we must do it by administering a triad of shocks to the mind. The best example is the advertising psychologist who stamps impressions upon our mind by the skilful use of large billboards, vivid colours and flashing neon lights.

Take a simple object, like a match, and attempt to visualize it with the intention of remembering 'match' as the first of five objects. Look at the match, close your eyes and mentally see it as having grown to the size of a telephone pole. Get a mental feeling of its enormous size. Now visualize this match as igniting and see the intense red of the flame and the sudden flare of ignition. At this point you have brought colour and motion into action, along with size, to stamp 'match' upon your memory.

Along with S.C.M. we use the better-known principle of association to permit retention of a series of visualizations. A link is established between each object through association.

Imagine a spark shooting off from the burning match and dropping on to the fluffy tail of a large white rabbit, who begins hopping around in an effort to snuff out his smouldering tail.

The rabbit starts brushing his teeth with a bright, yellow oversize toothbrush. Upon finishing he throws the toothbrush into a river which is rushing rapidly by. A deer comes down to drink from the river.

You should now find that you have effortlessly memorized five items, namely, match, rabbit, toothbrush, river and deer. It is as easy to link together twenty objects as it is five. The student is advised to experiment for himself.

CHAPTER SIX

REVITALIZATION

Yoga has always had very definite theories concerning mind and its potential use. The Yogi considers 'mind' as the highest evolvement of energy and this theory is not limited to just individual mind but is applied to the universe as a whole. Yoga suggests that the ultimate and original state of the universe is energy in the form of 'Cosmic Mind', which permeates everything conceivable and as a result man is said to be surrounded by 'mind', much as goldfish are surrounded by water.

When Cosmic Mind manifests itself, in building matter, the fundamental energy involved in such phenomena as cohesion, electricity, magnetism, etc., is termed *prana*, the basic kinetic energy of the universe. Such a cosmology naturally leads to the theory that since mind is all and a fundamental form of it is called *prana*, then each individual's mind should be able to control the *prana* or nervous energy within the physical body.

Contrary to Western science, Eastern science claims that nervous energy within the body may be increased, stored up and controlled at will by the mind.

This control energy (*prana*) is learned through mastery of *pranayama* (energy control) involving breathing exercises. It is postulated that the breath brings into the body *prana* as well as oxygen. This has lured many people into practising difficult, and sometimes dangerous, breathing techniques and very often they are disappointed with the apparent lack of pranic energy increase.

Raja Yoga holds the key which explains the apparent failure many people experience with *pranayama*. The key is concentration of the mind upon the body while performing *pranayama*. Just as the blood circulates through the body, so *Raja Yoga* teaches that the mind may be made to circulate consciously throughout the body. As blood is the vehicle of oxygen, so mind is the vehicle of *prana* and this is the whole secret of revitalizing and rejuvenating the body.

This practice of *Savasana* has taught you to carry the mind to any of the *Marmasthanani*, while polarization started you on the first experiments in controlling pranic energy. You are now ready for an effective rejuvenating technique that requires no mastery of a difficult *pranayama* exercise, but only the comfortable retention of breath, coupled with intense concentration upon the *Marmasthanani* or vital zones.

Specific Advantages

1. Increased oxygen absorption resulting in an increase in red blood cells.
2. The full inhalation required exercises the thoracic region, improving heart action and aiding return of venous blood to the heart.
3. *Prana* is consciously infused into the body and this results in a recharging of the nervous system.
4. A very specific antidote for quickly counteracting fatigue and exhaustion, both mental and physical.

Technique

1. Lie supine, with feet together, and hands, palms up, by your sides.
2. Inhale a slow, even, deep breath and hold it as soon as the lungs feel full. Retain the breath as long as is comfortable and without creating symptoms of strain.

3. While retaining the breath, mentally become aware of the feet (first vital zone) and visualize pranic energy radiating throughout that area and producing a tingle.

4. Slowly exhale, relaxing intensity of concentration.

5. Inhale again, retain and move to the next *Marmasthanani*, the shins, and repeat concentration.

6. Work up the body, retaining the breath and concentrating at each of the vital spots until you finish up at the head.

7. If necessary, go over the entire body several times until you feel a distinct glowing and tingling from toe to head.

Allow at least fifteen minutes for the exercise. In that time you should be able to go over the body three times or more, depending upon the retention period. The student should strive for fifteen seconds *kumbhak* or breath retention at the end of several months' practice. The key point is to become so consciously aware of each of the zones that your 'awareness' creates a tingling indicative of the successful infusion of *prana* into that zone.

Revitalization, when used in conjunction with other exercises, is excellent for bringing mind back from a deep state of introspection and monoideism, such as results from *Yoni Mudra*.

The student will discover that not only are physical results apparent in this technique, but also psychological effects appear in the form of a calm, relaxed attitude of mind. This is due to the respiratory process acting as a psychosomatic link between mind and body, as discussed in the chapter on *Yoni Mudra*.

The student must take note that the revitalization technique is definitely contra-indicated for those suffering from any form of heart disease.

CHAPTER SEVEN

LAYA YOGA THEORY

Laya Yoga is the science of unleashing latent energy hidden within the human nervous system.

As man has evolved from a primarily physically motivated animal to a mentally motivated animal, he has lost much of his physical strength and capacity for endurance. It could be that the strength and endurance of man's cave-dwelling ancestors still lie locked within his Central Nervous System (namely, the brain and spinal cord) in the form of potential energy. *Laya Yoga* is the key that attempts to unlock man's hidden energy reserves.

This latent energy is called *kundalini* and is symbolized by a snake coiled three-and-a-half times. The symbology of the snake gives us the secret implications of *kundalini*.

The snake has been a sexual symbol from time immemorial, and this tells us that *kundalini* is intimately connected with the sexual expression of man. Indeed sexual activity springs from the stream of *kundalini* force and is the most concrete example we have of a latent energy lying within us that has far-reaching effects in our life. The orgasm of sexual union is said to be similar to the trembling and bliss of *kundalini* rising.

This connection between sexual activity and *kundalini* has led to the development of two distinct schools of thought. The Tantra school teaches the rise and release of *kundalini* by using the physical act of intercourse as a channel for this energy to express itself through. The Yoga school teaches that sexual activity should be curtailed (*Bramacharya*), thus suppressing *kundalini* until the pressure becomes sufficiently strong for *kundalini* energy to force itself into arousal. Both schools of thought have half of the key in their respective viewpoints, and the result has been that both schools have thoroughly confused Westerners who have taken to practising the none-too-harmless exercises prescribed by each tradition.

Wisdom of Mental Control

The snake, as well as symbolizing the procreative urge, symbolizes wisdom – the wisdom of mental control. This is a hint that if such an energy as *kundalini* does exist, it may be released only through the mind exerting careful stimulation at the points where *kundalini* is most apt to manifest. The individual who would awaken or arouse *kundalini* without first gaining control of his mind, through *Raja Yoga* disciplines, would run the risk of mental illness.

The last point that should be brought to the student's attention concerns the fact that the snake is always shown as coiled. This coiling of a snake is preparation for striking out, and it is just so that *kundalini* lies within us compressed like a spring, and ready to charge from potential static energy into kinetic manifestation under the proper conditions. The coil of three represents the three states of energy (positive, negative and neutral), while the half coil represents *kundalini* as always on the verge of changing from static to kinetic manifestation.

It is taught in the East that just as the snake-charmer must first make himself immune to the poison of his snakes, so the student of *Laya Yoga* must prepare himself for the shock of arousing *kundalini* or suffer the consequences. It is also cautioned that the arousal of *kundalini* is easier than its control and subdual.

Process of Introspection

The ancient Yogis obtained their remarkable knowledge of the human body largely through a process of introspection. Through *Raja Yoga* they became so intensely aware of themselves that they internally 'felt', rather than 'saw', the major blood-vessels, nerves and organs. Out of such introspections grew a theory concerning the existence of certain *nadis* or psychic nerves through which *kundalini* could manifest.

The three most important of these astral channels were called *Ida, Pingala,* and *Shushumna. Ida* and *Pingala* are said to run up the left and right sides of the spine (corresponding with the sympathetic nerve ganglion on either side of the spine), while *Shushumna* runs between them in a position corresponding to the spinal cord.

Allegorically, *Shushumna* is said to represent the channel of 'Christ Consciousness' in us all which is kept vacant or 'crucified' by the emotions running rampant in *Ida* and *Pingala* (the two thieves hanging on either side of Christ).

Kundalini is stored at the base of the spine in the egg-shaped *kanda*, from which is said to emanate seventy-two thousand psychic nerves including *Ida, Pingala* and *Shushumna*. The object of *Laya Yoga* is to arouse *kundalini* and force it to ascend *Shushumna*, awakening various vital centres situated along the way, and finally uniting with the top centre, *Sahasrara*, where a union takes place between *kundalini shakti* (feminine or negative energy) and *siva shakti* (masculine or positive energy).

This concept may be taken as either symbolic or literal. Each 'chakra' or psychic centre, as it is touched by the ascending *kundalini*, has the God and Goddess dwelling within. This could be said to be the story of the union between the positive and negative aspects in our life, which takes place upon the ascent into spiritual consciousness.

Most commonly, it is taught that the human body contains seven major psychic centres, five situated along the spine and two found within the head. These centres are called *chakras* or *padmas*. *Chakra* means wheel and thus it is implied that these centres are moving or active. *Padma* means lotus and as a lotus, like any plant is something that grows, so the psychic centres are not fully developed in us but have yet to open their 'petals' into full bloom.

A psychic centre (*chakra* or *padma*) may be defined as a whirling vortex of energy situated at the conjunction point of the body and the mind.

The student may at first be repulsed by the idea of 'psychic centres', but if he considers that this teaching of *Laya Yoga* is in reality a 2,500-year-old theory only recently rediscovered by modern psychiatry as 'psychosomatic medicine', his attitude cannot help but be one of rational interest.

Each *chakra* is correlated with a major gland and a main nerve plexus within the body. By some coincidence, or method of analytical introspection now lost to us, the point where each *chakra* is located corresponds with the points in the body where psychosomatic tension most commonly manifests.

The Chakras

1. *Muladhara* means 'root support' and is situated at the base of the spine in the coccygeal region and is physically manifested through the gonads and the 'pelvic plexus'. Traditionally this *chakra* controls the sexual functions in humans and its malfunction at the psychic level would produce nymphomania and satyriasis. It is said to be responsible for such psychosomatic symptoms as impotency and frigidity.

2. *Swadhisthana* means 'one's own place'. All fluids in the body are balanced and controlled through this *chakra*. Physiologically related to the adrenal glands, kidneys and hypogastric plexus,

Swadhisthana has its root in the first few vertebrae of the sacral region. Malfunctioning of this *chakra* produces fluid disturbances such as oedema, blood poisoning, female troubles, obesity, etc.

3. *Manipura* or the 'gem city' emerges from the lumbar region of the spine and is physically evident as the solar plexus. The gland most often connected with *Manipura* is the pancreas. Some authorities also suggest the liver. The solar plexus (sun centre) has often been called the 'second brain' and its importance psychosomatically is readily appreciated by anyone who has ever suffered stomach cramps, 'butterflies', etc. Emotional tension first affects the solar plexus and sustained tension may be responsible for stomach ulcers, diabetes and even cancer.

4. *Anahata*, the centre of 'unstruck sound', comes out between the upper thoracic vertebrae and is related physiologically to the cardiac plexus and the thymus gland. Such psychosomatic disturbances as angina pectoris, palpitations, tachycardia, etc., may be logically related to this *chakra*.

5. *Vishuddha* or 'purity centre' is the last of the *chakras* rooted upon the spinal column (cervical region in this case). The thyroid gland and the pharyngeal plexus are associated with *Vishuddha* as its physical vehicles. Psychosomatic symptoms related to *Vishuddha* would include the depression often caused by thyroid malfunctioning and such speech difficulties as have a psychological rather than a physiological origin.

6. *Ajna* or the centre of 'non-knowledge' (indicative of something higher than human reason) is said to be situated between the eyebrows just about where the pituitary gland rests in the 'Turkis saddle'. *Ajna* is believed to be related to the nasociliary plexus. Tension, worry and anxiety are all said to arise from a disturbance of *Ajna*. This is interesting when we consider that the pituitary gland had been

named 'master gland' because of the effect its
secretions have upon the functioning of the other
ductless glands.

7. *Sahasrara chakra* means the 'thousand petalled'
centre. This is a reference to the thousands upon
thousands of brain cells contained within the
cerebrum, with which *Sahasrara* is related. The
gland connected with *Sahasrara* is the pineal – about
which we know too little.

Chakra Chart I

Sanskrit	English	Body Root	Plexus & Gland
Muladhara	'Root Support'	Coccyx	Pelvic Plexus
			Testes & Ovaries
Swadhisthana	'One's Own Place'	Sacral Vert. Navel (below)	Hypogastric Plexus Adrenal Glands
Manipura	'Gem City'	Lumbar Vert. Navel (above)	Solar Plexus Pancreas & Liver
Anahata	'Unstruck Sound'	Thoracic Vert. Heart Region	Cardiac Plexus Thymus Gland
Vishuddha	'Purity Centre'	Cervical Vert. Throat Area	Pharyngeal Plexus Thyroid Gland
Ajna	'Non-knowledge'	Nasion Between Eyes	Naso-ciliary Plexus Pituitary Gland
Sahasrara	'1,000-Petalled'	Bregma Top of Head	Cerebrum Pineal Gland

It is said that when *kundalini* rises up and unites
with *Suhasrara*, the resulting shock to the nervous
system awakens the pineal gland from its dormant
state and man finds himself possessed of *siddhis* or
psychic powers. These *siddhis* represent dormant
sensory faculties within man that have been lost
through disuse.

Australian aboriginals, for example, are still
capable of tracking a man by smell, much as a dog
does. The primitive native senses water in desert
areas and generally displays an acute sensitivity to
his environment which is lacking in his modernized
counterpart. His *siddhis*, like those of an animal,
have remained active through force of
circumstances.

I have by no means exhausted the material available on the theory of *Laya Yoga*, but have been concerned only with what is pertinent to the purpose of this book. Above all I have concentrated upon rationalizing all such theory into a more or less acceptable form.

Regarding the theory as a whole, the reader will readily discern two points:

1. The theory may be taken as an allegory of the ascent and transmutation of human consciousness into divine consciousness.

2. This ancient theory does contain material which has an undeniable implication and relationship with the hypothesis of modern psychosomatic medicine.

CHAPTER EIGHT

CHAKRA DHARANA

Mankind has always been aware of the existence of certain vital areas in the human body. The use to which the esoteric knowledge of these nerve zones was put varied from civilization to civilization.

The student will be interested to note that a correlation exists between the *chakras* of the Indian Yogi and the *kyushos* of the Japanese Judo expert. The seven most deadly *kyushos* (jiu-jitsu pressure points) taught in *Atemiwaza*, one of the esoteric branches of Judo, exactly correspond with the traditional positions of the seven chakras. While the Indian mind used this knowledge for spiritual and psychic purposes, the Japanese mind used the same knowledge for concrete physical purposes, namely, the induction of unconsciousness or even death (*Atemiwaza*) and the revival of those who had been so disabled (*kwappo*).

There is evidence to indicate that Judo originated in India, was taken up by the Tibetan monks as a means of self-defence (their religious vocation forbade the carrying of arms) and spread from Tibet to China, where it was picked up and developed by the Japanese in the fifteenth century. This is plausible if we also recall the migration and transmutation of Indian Buddhism to Japanese Zen.

It has been suggested by several modern schools of Yoga that the chakras, with their associated symbology, represent nothing more than a method of forcing the mind to concentrate upon the body.

COMPARISON CHART

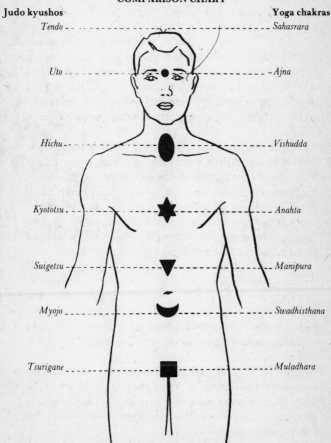

Judo kyushos		Yoga chakras
Tendo		Sahasrara
Uto		Ajna
Hichu		Vishudda
Kyototsu		Anahta
Suigetsu		Manipura
Myojo		Swadhisthana
Tsurigane		Muladhara

This may be so, especially when we consider that one of the literal meanings of the Sanskrit *Laya* is 'absorption'. Such absorption or concentration of the mind upon the body would lead to the 'opening' or harmonizing of the *chakras* and their respective psycho-physical functions.

This Eastern occult theory would be acceptable to the West if it could be proved that such concentration relaxed the psychosomatic tension that so often occurs in these vital areas. The author is certain that such concentration is helpful in dispersing tension at these very points and therefore feels justified in giving the technique of *Chakra Dharana*.

In the initial stages the mind is best trained by giving it something concrete to concentrate upon. This is the purpose of the elaborate symbology. Each *chakra* has a certain number of petals, each petal inscribed with a letter of the Sanskrit alphabet (this is for awakening the *chakra* through *Mantra Yoga*), an animal, a god and goddess, a geometrical form, a colour and a *Bija* or seed mantra.

All that will be necessary, for our purposes, will be a knowledge of the last three symbolic components, namely, colour, form, and *Bija* mantra. Students who are desirous of learning the full symbolic implications of each *chakra* are recommended to peruse Arthur Avalon's *The Serpent Power*.

The form and colour of the first five *chakras* represent the *tattwa* or element assigned to each. The *Bija* or seed *mantra* is the basic sound which groups or awakens the dormant energy of the individual *chakra*.

Symbology of Chakras

Muladhara: A yellow square representing *Prithivi*, the earth element. The *Bija* mantra is 'Lang'.

Swadhisthana: A silver crescent moon representing

Apas, the water element. *Bija* mantra is 'Vang' (changed 'Wang').

Manipura: A red triangle, apex down, representing *Tejas*, the fire element. *Bija* mantra is 'Rang'.

Anahata: A blue hexagon composed of two interlocked equilateral triangles representing *Vayu* or air element. *Bija* mantra is 'Yang'.

Vishuddha: A black or dark indigo, oval egg representing *Akasa* or ether. The *Bija* mantra is 'Hang'.

The procedure of *Chakra Dharana* begins with external *Dharana* and ends with internal *Dharana*. This type of concentration would be said to be a *Saguna* meditation or meditation upon concrete qualities as expressed through form and colour.

Chakra Chart 2

Chakra	Geometrical Form	Colour	Bija Mantra
Muladhara	Square	Yellow	'Lang'
Swadhisthana	Crescent Moon	Silver	'Vang'
Manipura	Triangle (Apex Down)	Red	'Rang'
Anahata	Hexagon	Blue	'Yang'
Vishuddha	Oval (Egg)	Black	'Hang'

Specific Advantages

1. Concentration and visualizing are improved.
2. Eastern occult theory states that this technique of concentration is the safest and most natural way of gently awakening and harmonizing the 'Psychic Centres'.
3. Relaxation of psychosomatic tension should accrue from steady practice.

Preparation

Reference to the diagram entitled *Tattwa Yantras* will provide a clear picture of the symbolical representation of each *chakra* through its *tattwa* or quality. To produce models of these *yantras* suitable for use, the student will require a selection of yellow, silver, red, blue, and black drawing paper such as is commonly given to children for cutting and pasting.

With a ruler and compasses construct each geometrical figure upon the correct colour of paper. Thus the square is inscribed upon yellow, the crescent upon silver, the triangle (apex down) upon red, the hexagon upon blue and the oval upon black.

It is now a simple procedure to cut out each pattern and paste it upon the centre of a large square of black paper (with the exception of the black oval, which needs a white background). The final result is a set of five *Tattwa Yantras* which may be affixed to the wall for the technique of external *Chakra Dharana*.

Technique

1. Sit in a meditative posture or in a chair, with the room lit by a candle.
2. Place before you the yellow square *tattwa* of *Muladhara Chakra*, with the candle on one side so that the diagram is illuminated.
3. Fix the gaze upon the centre of the square and audibly (*udgita*) intone the *Bija* mantra 'Lang'.
4. Continue this procedure for three to five minutes, attempting to occupy your mind completely with the yellow square and the *Bija* mantra.
5. Close your eyes and mentally visualize the yellow square while silently repeating (*audgita*) the *Bija* mantra.
6. In the final step, move the *tattwa* symbol down into its appropriate spot on your own spine. (In this case visualize the yellow square as at the base of your spine.) Continue concentration as long as possible.

CHAKRA TATTWA YANTRAS

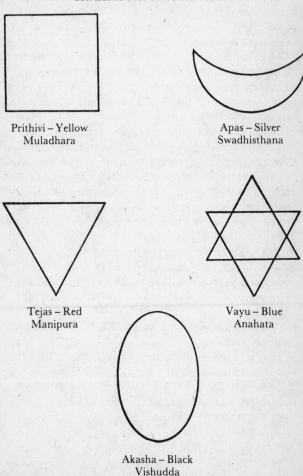

Prithivi – Yellow
Muladhara

Apas – Silver
Swadhisthana

Tejas – Red
Manipura

Vayu – Blue
Anahata

Akasha – Black
Vishudda

Practice Routine

The technique of *Chakra Dharana* should be practised for ten minutes or more each day. Begin with *Muladhara Chakra* the first day, *Swadhisthana Chakra* the second day and so on, doing each *chakra* in turn until you return to *Muladhara* and start the cycle over again.

After the first two or three weeks the student may dispense with external *Dharana* in the form of concentration upon a *tattwa* diagram and may proceed with just internal *Dharana* upon the *chakra* symbols within the body.

With practice the student will produce a sensation of actual physical stimulation by mentally moving the *tattwa* symbol down into its proper position along the spine and concentrating upon the area. The yellow square of *Muladhara* should be visualized as at the base of the spine; the silver crescent of *Swadhisthana* is two inches below the naval; the red triangle of *Manipura* is about three inches above the navel, level with the pit of the stomach; the blue hexagram of *Anahata* should be visualized as level with the heart; and the black egg of *Vishuddha Chakra* is level with the Adam's apple.

In essence, internal *Chakra Dharana* is the familiar tantric technique of 'internalization' of gods, colours, forms, etc.

The technique of concentration upon the sixth and seventh *chakras, Ajna* and *Sahasrara*, is unnecessary for the student at this stage and hence is deemed outside the scope of this book.

CHAPTER NINE

SOLAR PLEXUS CHARGING

The student has now reached the point where he may be introduced to pure *Laya* technique. I must, however, warn the student that the material presented in this chapter is beyond rationalization, and other than offering my apologies for teaching a seemingly high speculative practice, I may only hope that the student will progress to the point where he is in a position to prove the postulations set forth, to his own satisfaction.

Advanced *Laya* exercises are directly concerned with the awakening of *chakras* and the arousal of *kundalini* to the point where the practitioner experiences definite subjective and objective changes taking place within the body.

Closely Guarded Secrets

The *kriyas* or techniques, bringing about the ascent of *kundalini* up *Shushumna*, are amongst the most closely guarded secrets of *Laya Yoga*. My own knowledge of these methods was given to me in confidence by my teacher and, of the six exercises, I am only permitted to pass on the first phase, termed 'Solar Plexus Charging'. I should remark that even if the aspiring student had access to the mechanics of the five succeeding *kriyas*, it would be of little value, as the degree of concentrative ability required to bring about results would, in all probability, be beyond his present stage of development.

Just as certain pathological conditions produce

distinct · symptoms permitting an accurate diagnosis, so the arousal of *kundalini* is traditionally marked by specific symptoms. The first definite indication that latent nerve energy is being successfully released into the body is the appearance of psychic heat.

At first this is subjective and the student simply becomes aware of warm currents running up and down the spine and circulating in the region of the solar plexus. Later the currents become hot, and anyone passing his hand along the student's spine will feel distinct heat waves emanating from whatever *chakra* region the *kundalini* energy has ascended to. As *kundalini* rises, the heat waves move from the base of the spine to the top cervical region.

Tibetan Yogins make particular use of this psychic heat in a process called *tumo*, mastery of which permits wandering naked in the snow-covered Himalayas.

Specific Advantages

1. The solar plexus storehouse (*manipura chakra*) overflows with pranic energy and this surplus is automatically distributed wherever needed.
2. The arousal of *kundalini* and the resulting heat produced will entirely change the student's attitude towards 'cold'. Once it is experienced, the body never really becomes cold again.
3. The mind becomes deeply absorbed in the exercise as the production of heat increases.

Technique

1. Lie supine, head north, feet south, in a semi-dark room, with the legs folded in *Sukhasana* (as if you had fallen backwards while in *Sukhasana*) and the hand clasped over the solar plexus.
2. On a slow, even inhalation, visualize warm, golden pranic energy being drawn in through the head (as in polarization) and down the body into

the thighs and lower abdominal region, where it is prevented from escaping by your crossed feet and is therefore stored.

3. On a slow, even exhalation, bring the accumulated prana up and around the solar plexus in a series of clockwise circles (as if you had a clock dial, the size of a dinner plate, centred over the navel with twelve o'clock at the chest and six o'clock at the groin).

4. Making as many circles as possible, while exhaling, concentrate upon feeling an internal heat develop with each visualization of an energy sweep around the solar plexus.

The exercise should be carried out for never less than fifteen minutes. Once the student succeeds he will be surprised to realize that the inner psychic heat produced is not the result of 'self-hypnosis'. The mechanics of the exercise, when analyzed, reveal several interesting theories peculiar to Yoga.

Yoga physiology maintains that the hands and feet are terminals through which the body throws off psychic energy in the form of Prana. The crossing of the feet and interlocking of the hands short-circuit the escape of *prana* and results in an additional source of energy for Solar Plexus charging. The crossing of the feet relaxes sexual tension as well and thus another possible source of energy waste is prevented. It is with this *kriya* that we realize the need of a new physiology capable of explaining the release of hitherto unsuspected energy reserves.

Once the induction of psychic heat is accomplished the student will find his mind becoming more and more absorbed in the performance of this *kriya*. He will come to understand the *Laya* truly means absorption and rhythm such as can be found only within the eternity of his own consciousness – the link with Universal Consciousness.

CHAPTER TEN

YOGIC POWER FLOWS

The *siddhis* represents supra-sensual and supra-sensory controls bestowed upon the Yoga adept as the result of *sadhana* or practice. Mcdonell's Sanskrit Dictionary defines *siddhi* as 'hitting of a mark, accomplishment, performance, fulfilment, complete attainment, success, getting the better of, cure (of a disease), attainment of one's aims, success, fortune, personal perfection entailing the acquisition of supernatural powers, magical power (magic is the art of causing changes to occur in conformity with the will of *Itcha Shakti*), efficacy, efficiency, skill, demonstration.'

The demonstration of *siddhis* is a by-product of one-pointedness (*Ekagrata*) and neural equilibrium (*Yoga*), through years of technique (*Kriya*).

Mind-Body Durability

Over the decades a constant source of personal excitement for me has been the exploration of my own mind-body durability against the fundamental elements of nature; fire, blood, steel. Man is conditioned from infancy to fear fire, blood and steel and the conquest of such fear is symbolical of the ascent of spirit over matter.

For my own mastery I am indebted to a series of adepts, both Eastern and Western. Indeed, in India some of the secret *siddha Yoga Kriya* is inherited from father to son and may be passed down generation after generation. Immunity to fire and pain is not a trick in the sense of 'sleight-of-hand' or 'mirrors' but rather the ultimate *confidence* trick.

Confidence literally means a mental state of togetherness (Greek prefix *con*) in perfect trust, faith and fidelity (Latin *fides*) to one's own true self – in short, 'trance-consciousness' or transcendence of the little self which is so habitually filled with doubts and insecurities.

Even a momentary lapse of such *confidence* (Yoga) during a demonstration can mean a trip to the hospital or morgue for the foolhardy and unenlightened. The three *chakras* below the diaphramic partition give control over fire, blood and steel, as follows.

Muladhara Chakra
Opening of *Muladhara* gives power over all the elements of the earth, including metals (particularly steel) and the earth part of man or flesh.

After the opening of *Muladhara,* pain control becomes a reality with the skewering of the flesh, spiking, the oft-joked about 'bed of nails' (everyman's life!) and ultimate crucifixion preceded by the crown of thorns (opening the *Sahasrara chakra*) producing At-One-Ment.

Swadhisthana Chakra
Mastery of the blood flow in the Deha or physical body of the yogi arises with the opening of this force centre. Vaso-constriction and vaso-dilation of the arterioles at will and even cessation of capillary oozing occurs. Stigmata or the percolation of blood through the skin to the outside environment can also be demonstrated.

Swadhisthana is the fluid control point for the entire system. With the opening of *Swadhisthana*, the inherent 'swami' or water-walker of each man and woman emerges.

Manipura Chakra
This is the centre of the salamander, fire-walker and fire-breather, whose inner life is sustained by the sustenance of the primal heat element. The fire-walkers of North India who tread across beds of glowing embers, the Pacific islanders who walk upon white-hot stones, employ the Manipura chakra, as do the lickers of white-hot bars.

So-called 'fire-eaters' unwittingly use the *Manipura chakra* in conjunction with the *Anahata chakra* (air or *pranayama* centre) to perform their feats.

Simultaneous mastery of earth, water and fire with subsequent immunity to pain and searing of flesh by heat, is accomplished through juggling of the forces inherent in the first three *chakras* blossoming upon the tree of life. Classical demonstrations include dipping the hands into boiling water, boiling oil, molten lead (lead melts at three times the temperature of boiling water), and molten steel – also bathing in and drinking these substances.

Tongue Piercing
In the Hindu tradition, *siddhi* rituals are a religious act of supplication to the goddess Durga for Karmic purification. All ceremonies begin by piercing the tongue with a dirty, unsterile spike or skewer. This results in the reflex awakening of the *Swadhisthana chakra*, permitting 'fire to be fought with water'.

Just transfixing the tongue alone is no petty feat, for although the sensitivity to pain varies in different body areas, the tongue – along with genitals, eardrums and the eye cornea – shares the distinction of being one of the most painful and sensitive regions in the body. (Remember the last time you bit your tongue?)

Hindu Torture Ritual

A group of medical doctors investigating Hindu torture ritual in Fiji stated:

> The piercing of the tongue, however, is a different matter. It is a very sensitive organ. The participants maintain that no pain was felt when the tongue was pierced, and that no bleeding took place. There was certainly no sign of either. Whereas the absence of blood during skin puncturing can perhaps be explained in other terms, the piercing of the tongue cannot. It is blood-filled and tender. There can be no doubt that the normal bleeding reaction, as well as the normal pain reaction, was successfully overcome by whatever processes are involved in the rituals.
>
> (*Holy Torture in Fiji*, Pacific Publications, Sydney, Australia).

An ounce of practice is worth a pound of theory, one picture is worth a thousand words – one demonstration a year is worth eleven theoretical lectures. The purpose of unleashing psycho-physiological power through the *siddhis* is to create a psychic shock in the witnesses, so that a momentary realization of life's potential is experienced. Such demonstrations provide TAN-gible proof of the TRA-nscendence possible through TAN-TRA.

Tantric Sexuality

In 1975 my book *Sexual Occultism* was published by Llewellyn Publications (P.O. Box 3383, St Paul, MN 55165, U.S.A.). A revised edition was produced by Compendium Pty Ltd (R.S.D. Birregurra South, Victoria, Australia 3242) in 1977. The Introduction states: 'It is my profound hope that encouragement will be given to all, through this book, for utilizing the sexual dimension as a key unlocking joyous power.'

In these purportedly enlightened times let me make several flat statements at the very outset of this chapter.

All Yoga is really derived from *Tantra*. Gurudev Satyananda says: 'Yoga is an offshoot of Tantra.' (*Tantra – Yoga Panorama*). The scholastic proof of this is outside the scope of this chapter but we will deal with it another time.

Westerners (who love gossip about sexual matters) equate *Tantra* with *sexuality*. This is incorrect, as sexual considerations form but a small fragment of the total tantric teaching and indeed sexual references are sparse in the Tantra Shastras – most of which have not yet been translated into European languages. However the attitude in *Tantra* to sexual expression is one of liberation and reality rather than repression or suppression.

Quoting my friend Dr Sinha (Director of the India Institute of Yoga, Patna) writing in his book *Yoga, Meaning and Values:* 'According to Yoga, sex is not an evil nor a sin. It is neither degrading nor weakening. On the contrary, according to Tantra Yoga, *sex is regarded as generative of vitality, energy and power, and also as a harmonizer of the senses.*'

The zoologist Desmond (*The Naked Ape*) Morris ascribes ten distinct purposes to sexual experience. Beginning with *procreative sex* (the most primal of sexual functions – anyone who limits sexual activity to procreation needs a psychiatrist!) his enumeration includes *physiological sex* (relief), *occupational sex* (anti-boredom device), *tranquillizing sex* (anxiety reducing), and *status sex* (aggression release), as well as five other categories. Using his brilliant analysis of sexual function from a biological viewpoint, we could add three further dimensions to sexuality which derive directly from tantric wisdom.

Sex for Consciousness Expansion

An orgasm tends to automatically illuminate the nervous system in a way traditionally described as 'awakening *kundalini*'. Nearly everyone can learn to deepen, prolong and enhance this state, through some types of tantric methodology, using the orgasm as a springboard to transcendence.

Sex for E.S.P. Development
Sexual activity promotes sensory hyperacuity or 'sensory awareness' (at least it should!) Tantric Sexual *Sadhana* induces profound experiences of E.S.P. or Extra-*Sensual*-Perception, converting the whole skin into one extensive, massive, genital organ. (Etymologically one meaning of the Sanscrit root 'tan' is 'to extend').

Humans are so 'out of touch' with their own bodies that few ever even experience the two erogenic zones in each hand which are tantric chakras. Those who open up the full potential of the five sensory gates through Tantric Sexual *Sadhana* will immeasurably speed their 'psychic' development.

Sex for 'Positive Thinking'
Sexual arousal, culminating in a climax, is the key to attitude-changing or 'self-hypnosis'. The English psychiatrist William Sargeant (*Battle for the Mind*) rediscovered the tantric secret that a sexually aroused human is hypersuggestible. Correct use and knowledge of this (sometimes called 'sex magic') allows an individual to consciously inculcate his unconscious with life-affirming – rather than life-negating – attitudes.

Sexual Terminology
Etymology and semantics, coupled with psycholinguistics, reveal the esoteric and arcane function that erotic impulse serves in the human organism. The following are a few examples taken from my book *Sexual Occultism*.

Climax The word, which we use as a term for the desirable culmination of sexual stimulation, comes from the Greek *klimax* meaning a 'ladder' or 'staircase to heaven'. It indicates the inner significance of sexuality as a spiritual path. This is unconsciously implicit in the joke that a 'run' in nylon stockings or pantihose is a 'ladder to heaven'.

Clitoris From Greek through to Latin, as in *clavis*, a 'key'. That part of the female vulva which unlocks her nervous system the way a key unlocks a door. The central genital pushbutton for ecstasy.

Consummate Used in the contemporary sense of completing a marriage through intercourse. The original Latin root is replete with the significance of the esoteric object of intercourse, for 'consummate' is to bring to completion (Yoga) or perfection, make perfect (*siddhi*), highest, topmost, utmost, and the 'crown of'. (The object of tantric intercourse is to open *Sahasrara* or the 'crown' *chakra*).

Create From the Sanskrit root *kr* meaning 'to make', through to Latin as *creare*, implying production, growing, to bring into existence. The close relationship between sexual fecundity and mental originality is demonstrated by our use of the word 'create' to denote both creation of life and artistic creativity.

The birth of ideas is an analogue to physical birth. We interchange words like 'conceiving' and 'conception', using them both for either physical pregnancy or mental agility. We also speak of a 'fertile woman' and a 'fertile imagination'.

Occult psychology views the mind as divided into the masculine active consciousness and the feminine passive unconscious. The art of mental creation is an alchemical process of impregnating the unconscious mind with a seed or germinal idea, grasped by consciousness but ejaculated into the deeper unconscious realms for incubation. Gestation continues in the unconscious womb until the sudden birth of the idea as a 'flash' or 'inspiration' which emerges – fully formed – into consciousness.

Orgasm Found in English, through French and Latin, from two closely related Greek roots; *orgio*, a sacred rite, sacrifice (of semen?) ceremony in the early Graeco-Roman mysteries celebrating the feast of Dionysius or Bacchus, hence our expression 'an orgy'. The second related root is *orgasio*, meaning 'to swell' with ardent desire, passion (expansion of the auric field in the way a balloon is over-inflated), 'to burst'; namely, an experience of such intense excitement that the ego is momentarily fragmented, producing a nameless-formless inner state.

Venerate Allied to the Sanskrit *van*, to love or honour, but directly taken from the Latin *vener*, to revere and love. Related words from the same Latin stem are 'venerable', 'venereal' and 'Venus' (the Roman goddess of love). To venerate is to recognize the sexual parts as truly worthy objects of our adoration and awe.

In conclusion, let us realize that – contrary to popular belief and teachings – the sexual dynamics of life have by no means been neglected as a source of spiritual *Sadhana* in the Indian *Tantra Yoga*. In particular, the tantrist worships woman as divinity personified and sexual *Sadhana* is an oblation to the eternal female. It is the Mother Goddess sustaining manifest existence as eternal *Shakti* who is incarnate in each woman.

Secret Science of Hand Gestures

The word *mudra* (as applied to hand positions) has the multiple meanings of 'sign', 'symbol' and 'gesture'. *Mudra* in this context is a secret sign language sending a message from the body to the mind via the nervous system and from conscious to unconscious spheres of existence.

A simple example of this occurs when practising *Savasana* (deep relaxation pose) lying supine with the palms placed uppermost in *Shunya Mudra* or the 'empty gesture', signalling the mind to become receptive (empty). *Shunya Mudra* is that universal open-handed sign 'I give in'; 'trust', 'surrender', 'relaxation', 'letting go'.

Mudra also means 'a seal', 'short cut' and 'short circuit' – indicating an actual physiological basis for effects of hand gestures by closing or uniting certain neurological reflex points which terminate on the cutaneous surface of the hands.

The famous *Gnana* (pronounced *G-yan*) *Mudra* formed by joining thumb and forefinger, leaving the remaining three fingers gently extended, demonstrates the anatomical, neurological and psychological principles of *Mudra*. *Gnana Mudra* means literally 'the wisdom gesture'; the Sanskrit *Gnana* giving rise to Greek *gnosis*, through into English as 'knowing'. He who meditates in *Gnana Mudra* affirms a subsuming of all the wisdom of the universe, thus placing the mind automatically in an optimum state for higher consciousness. Why?

The Thumb: Man
Let us begin with the thumb, which is the digit symbolizing man; finite, limited, but at the top of the evolutionary phylogenetic scale as 'the greatest of beasts'. The characteristic of a *human* ('humus' or earth creature) is his developed mind (Sanskrit *manas*) coupled with a tool-making capacity or manual dexterity excelling that of all other animals.

This tool-making ability is due to the anatomical development of the 'saddle joint' at the base of the thumb where it joins the wrist. The 'saddle joint' allows the thumb to be placed firmly in apposition to all the other fingers, thus permitting manual flexibility and grasping to a degree not found in other mammals and primates.

The Index Finger: God

The index finger (so called because we instinctively 'index' or classify all creation outside ourselves by pointing with this foremost or 'forefinger' digit) represents *God*, the absolute sea of cosmic energy that is infinite, limitless and eternal.

Uniting the thumb with the index finger forms a circle in which finite, limited man is linked with the infinite, unlimited absolute. The circle is a *(w)hole*, being both absolute zero and utter completeness. Pascal, the seventeenth-century French theologian, defined God as a circle whose circumference is nowhere and centre everywhere.

It is incorrect to say 'God' *exists*; only man exists and the moment something exists it is already limited by form and name (*Namarupa*). God *subsists* and *persists* but never *exists*.

Principle of Trinity

When forming the *Gnana Mudra* gesture, the remaining three fingers represent the principle of trinity in major world religions. Christianity conceives the Father, Son and Holy Ghost. Ancient Egypt immortalized Horus, Isis and Osiris as a triplicity, while Hinduism rests upon a tripod of Brahma, Vishnu and Shiva.

The gods and goddesses of theology esoterically represent – not persons – but rather forces responsible for the manifestation of all creation. Existence is the result of an interplay of three forces: positive, negative, neutral; male, female, hermaphrodite, the sun (positive), the earth (receptive), and the moon (neutralizing transformer).

In assuming *Gnana Mudra* for meditation and *pranayama* you have telegraphed to your unconscious that you possess all that can be known about life, yourself and the universe.

Man is an organism who has developed an intimate relationship between his hands and brain, hence whatever he does with his hands affects, through his nervous system, the cerebral cortex and the associated conscious and unconscious layers of mind.

In a general context all hand *mudra* is a special category of body language which is instinctual and universal amongst both primitive and civilized races.

Hastha Mudras

A very interesting group of *mudras* are referred to as *Hastha mudras*, which automatically gesture the breath into the abdominal rib cage or collar-bone area of the lungs. These special hand positions readjust the relationship between the pelvic girdle and the shoulder girdle in such a manner that expansion of desired lobes of the lungs occurs in preference to alternate possibilities.

For the beginner in *Hatha Yoga* the *Hastha Mudra* technique is a dramatic introduction to yoga breathing or *pranayama*, bestowing breath control upon the merest tyro. At any given moment the position of our hands exerts a subtle but profound influence which actually determines the manner in which we breathe.

Mudra is the psychic science relating hand and brain, gesture and state of consciousness. Following the Hermetic axiom 'as above so below', our finger movements betray our inner state at point-instant in time; hence the nervous drumming with finger tips of the agitated or eager are described as 'having itchy fingers'. Conscious assumption of ritual *Mudra* reverses this psychosomatic arc, moulding mind, breath and body into the willed or desired state required as a prelude to ultimate inner life experience.

CHAPTER ELEVEN

YOGA AND THE WEST

Yoga is the world's oldest and most effective method of achieving total mental and physical health. The whole person is included in Yoga, all aspects of the 'self'. What do we mean? The United Nations World Health Organisation has defined health as 'A condition of mental, physical and social well-being and not merely the absence of disease.' This statement is in perfect accordance with the goal and aims of Yoga in general.

Yoga is evolutionistic in approach. Western science, from the time of Darwin, has accepted the principle that all living creatures have evolved their physical features over a period of time on the basis of adapting to change and survival of the fittest. In terms of the human animal, Western biologists consider that the body is fully mature and ceases growth around the age of 25. But what of the mind?

Self-realization

Yoga has always taught that man's growth does not cease with maturity of the physical body. Each of us contains an unlimited potential mental and psychic growth affecting our personalities. The individual who evolves wholly as a person will eventually experience a mental state that is called self-realization in Yoga. He or she will become fully aware of the inner possibilities and richness of the mind. Western psychologists belonging to what is sometimes called 'Cognitive Schools' call this state 'self-actualization'.

Yoga is a technique that makes a better person of a Christian, Hindu, atheist, socialist and agnostic alike. Better people make better communities, better communities make better nations, and better nations make a better world.

The Indian Rope Trick

Who has not heard of the Indian rope trick? This legendary feat of Oriental magic involves the magician throwing a coil of rope into the air. Suddenly the rope hangs erect and suspended by magic. A small boy appears, climbs to the top of the rope, and vanishes into thin air.

Everyone has heard of this trick but no one has ever witnessed it. Why? Because the trick is not a feat but an allegory or story about your life and mine. The magician is the creative power of mind. The boy is the unrealized or immature self. The rope is an astral umbilical cord, *Sushumna* or Jacob's ladder, giving access to heaven or the sky. ('Heaven' is a state of mind). The whole legend is a statement about how man may utilize Yoga to rise above the earth or materialism, escaping the pettiness of ego and limited self to find freedom of mind and body.

The Essence of Hatha

The object of all Yoga is to induce a harmonious release of energy at the intellectual, emotional and physical levels of man's being. In *Hatha Yoga* the two syllables *Ha* (Sun) and *Tha* (Moon) refer to the inherent duality of all living organisms expressed as expansion and contraction, relaxation and tension, reflected right down to the cellular levels of metabolic building up (anabolism) and breaking down (catabolism).

In terms of the gross energy known to Western science, *Hatha Yoga* practice achieves a correct balance of using sugar and oxygen for energy and throwing out carbon dioxide and water as breakdown products of this burning.

The effect of all *asanas* or poses in *Hatha* can be summed up once the principle that 'nature tolerates no empty spaces' is understood. All twisting and bending of the body through *asanas* produces an internal compression massage of the tightly packed body organs, releasing vitality just as a sponge (body organ, for example, liver) can be cleansed by immersing in a basin of water (the body and circulating fluids) and systematically squeezing and releasing it.

Every student of the philosophical life should find at least a few minutes daily for some of the classical life-affirming poses of Hatha. In Lawrence Durrell's *Justine*, Balthazar – the cabalistic physician – comments: '...after all the work of the philosophers on his soul and the doctors on his body, what can we say we really know about man? That he is, when all is said and done, just a passage for liquids and solids, *a pipe of flesh*.' (My emphasis).

The efficacy of *Hatha Yoga* maintains the 'pipe of flesh' as the perfected vehicle of expression (*Tha*) for the enlightened consciousness (*Ha*).

Handling Emergency Situations

Maturity as a yoga teacher may be judged by how efficiently you handle emergency situations in the class. The moment an incident arises, if possible isolate the student requiring attention and keep the remainder occupied under the supervision of a senior student.

A Faint When a person falls or sags unconscious to the ground and rapidly recovers.

A Fit The collapse of a person who falls unconscious and then jerks or twitches. (Most commonly epileptic).

A Fall When the student slips or trips and lands

on the floor, often in balance exercises. When this
occurs, consider the possibility that he may have
struck his head when landing, particularly if he
seems dull after the incident and fails to get up.
Although you may think he overbalanced, always
ask if this was because he felt strange, weak, giddy
or sick.

Students attending Yoga classes on an empty
stomach and after a working day, may be
predisposed to giddiness and fainting. Any healthy
person can, under the right circumstances, faint.
All that is necessary is sufficient retardation of
blood flow to the brain (student with low blood-
pressure comes suddenly upright after inverted
posture), or lack of adequate oxygen (anaemic
student in crowded class who breathes in shallow
fashion), or lack of adequate blood-sugar level for
energy metabolism (diabetic student or exhausted
student who has not eaten, faints after *Surya
Namaskar* – having suddenly lowered the blood-
sugar level through muscular exertion).

Fainting in Various Circumstances

Fainting occurs in a variety of circumstances – high
temperature (air-condition or ventilate studio, if
possible), crowding (ideally never have more than
12 to a class), emotional shocks such as a fright or
sight of an accident or blood.

Susceptibility to fainting varies, some people
having a high threshold requiring very strong
stimulus, but given the right circumstances, anyone
– fit or not – will faint. In sickness, fainting will be
precipitated by the same factors as in health.
However, the stimulus required will be much less,
thus Yoga students should stay away from classes
when ill, even with influenza.

Since fainting is a reduction of brain-blood flow,
nature's method of causing unconsciousness and
falling to the ground is, in fact, self-correcting.

Blood-flow to the brain rapidly returns in the prone position and the victim recovers.

If consciousness does not return shortly, something more serious than a simple faint has occurred. Concussion (or actual damage to the brain in the cranial cavity) may be indicated by a continuing stuporous or comatose condition, vomiting shortly after, and unequal eye-pupil size. All those fainting and/or striking their heads on the floor should be recommended for examination by a medical doctor. Other students should witness the recommendation.

A Stupor A semi-conscious state in which the individual is prone, appears unconscious, but responds to strong pain stimulus or auditory stimulus such as pinching the skin or shouting the student's name. (In *Varami* we alter the psychic and emotional state by blowing sharply in the student's ear, particularly to bring him or her out of trance or deep meditation).

A Coma A profound unconsciousness, usually due to a drug overdose, poison, or severe organic brain damage. A quick and safe trick used by the Japanese police to differentiate between a stupor and a coma is to press a thin coin, key, or other thin, blunt object strongly under the thumb nail.

If the condition is a stupor, arousal will be almost instantaneous, as the nerve fibres conducting pain impulses are exquisitely sensitive under the fingernails, inducing cortical alertness. (Ever heard of bamboo splinters judiciously inserted under the nails? The Chinese have found them marvellous for facilitating memory when people seem to be having difficulty answering questions).

Frequently the student has warning signs of an impending faint; these include a feeling that things are receding far away, the world is becoming strangely quiet. He may go pale, yawn, begin to perspire (particularly if hypoglycaemic or suffering from lowered blood sugar), with beads of sweat or droplets bursting out on the forehead. (Treat by getting sugar, candy and so on, into him immediately). Fellow students may notice these signs.

Let him assume the hare posture, prone with head low and hips or buttocks high to restore normal circulation to the brain; or place him supine with feet propped up at a right angle against a wall.

In the case of a full faint, quickly observe the following points:

1. See that there is no obstruction to the neck from tight clothes.
2. Check that false teeth are not loose in the mouth or have not fallen back into the throat.
3. See that the student is not in a position that is harmful or dangerous to himself, for example, with one arm bent at an unusual angle under the body.

Acupuncture Resuscitation Method

Place the student supine and – rapidly grasping his heels – firmly raise his legs *abruptly* and *sharply* to a distinct right angle with the floor, then quickly smack the soles of his feet with the fingers of one hand, while holding both feet upright with the other hand. You are stimulating a point we call Kidney I, which is very popular with the Chinese for reviving victims of drowning and initiating the cardio-respiratory cycle in cases of syncope.

In Western medical practice, obstetricians have now abandoned the routine of slapping the buttocks of the newborn to stimulate breathing. They have discovered that if this is done carelessly, spinal damage can sometimes result. The preferred method is to grasp the infant upside-down by the ankles with one hand and slap the soles of his feet with the other. Raising the legs suddenly at right angles reverses venous stasis in lower limbs and rushes blood out of the limbs, through the abdominal cavity into the chest and then to the brain.

As the person recovers, persuade him not to get up for a while, as a faint may recur if there is too rapid a return to the normal upright posture. (*N.B.* Placing a person upright who is still in a dead faint will induce an epileptic fit, as the motor cells of the cortex will then be so severely oxygen-deprived that they will discharge erratically, causing tonic and clonic contractions of the muscular-skeletal system).

There are no after-effects of a simple faint, unless the patient is held upright while he is unconscious. This has occasionally happened when a person in a crowd cannot fall or a person sitting upright in a dental chair faints.

Bhastrika (the bellows), *Bhujangasana* (the cobra) and *Simhasana* (the lion pose) may all induce fainting in students with organic abnormalities or low blood-pressure.

In Yoga we have a special secret science of 'fainting' called *Murcha*. This induces ecstasy and a state beyond *Nama-rupa* (name-form) which is egoless. There are 44 such *Murchas*, which alter the blood chemistry and the blood flow to the brain, as well as affecting the activity of the autonomic nervous system. My own master of this hidden science was Swami Shantananda, who initiated me as Swami Ashimananda at Birla Mundir Temple, New Delhi, in 1960.

CHAPTER TWELVE

MEDITATION AND INNER BEING

Yoga students are often confused about meditation. The Oxford dictionary states that to meditate is 'having in mind to do or make, to ponder over, indulge in thought.' This definition gives the impression that meditation is an active, ongoing process of the mind with many thoughts, like fish, swimming through the stream of consciousness. The implication is that meditation is a form of thinking; namely, a problem-solving activity. Nothing could be further from the truth!

The word 'meditation' is inadequate to describe the higher mental states sought in Yoga. The object of Yoga exercises is to induce a state of mental quietness, of tranquillity which is far removed from pondering or indulging in active thought. A state of 'no-thought' better describes the result of Yoga.

The ancient author of the world's first known text of yoga was Patanjali, who defined Yoga as stilling the mind, making motionless the consciousness, and suppressing emotional fluctuations.

Eight Progressive Steps

Patanjali lucidly outlined eight progressive steps to be followed by those seeking experience of Yoga mental states. His system is termed *Ashtanga Yoga;* literally the eight limbs or branches leading to absolute integration of the self through fusion of the personality in trance consciousness.

The first two phases of *Ashtanga Yoga* are the *Yama* and *Niyama*, comprising ten rules of conduct or behaviour for the student desiring a unified life. Western scholars have confused the *Yama* and *Niyama* precepts with the Ten Commandments of Moses, not understanding that the concept of sin or punishment is foreign to Yoga. *Karma*, the law of action and reaction, is impartial in Eastern teaching. *Karma* is the psychological equivalent of Newton's physical law that for every action there must be an equal and opposite reaction. The *Yama-Niyama* practices are based upon a knowledge of *Karma*, and unlike the Ten Commandments, are devoid of moral or ethical meaning.

For example, '*Ahimasa* is the *Yama* of observing non-violence towards all creatures.' This dictum is based on the knowledge that we pay for violent acts or feelings by the loss of our peace of mind. Mental agitation precludes higher psychic states.

Santosha, the cultivation of contentment, is the *Niyama* rule of living in present time without brooding over the past or day-dreaming about the future. Living in present time conserves the psychic energy needed for meditation or super-consciousness.

The aim of these precepts is purely the maintenance of mental hygiene.

Yamas
1. *Ahimsa;* Non-violence.
2. *Satya;* Truth. Maintaining a lie wastes energy and disrupts internal states.
3. *Asteya;* Non-stealing. We have a right only to that which we have earned.
4. *Brahmacharya;* Sexual expansion.
5. *Aparigraha;* Non-possession or detachment from materialism.

Niyamas
1. *Saucha*; Purity of the physical body and freedom from toxic wastes.

2. *Santosha;* Contentment. Living in the eternal 'now'.

3. *Tapas;* Indifference to extremes or external change.

4. *Svadhyaya;* Self-development. When we cease learning we begin to die.

5. *Ishvarapranidhana;* Devotion to the philosophical life.

The third stage of Patanjali's classical system is *Asana*, meaning any position which is relaxed and sustained, allowing the body to be held motionless while mental silence is sought. Body activity is linked with mental states and the object of *Asana* is to reduce the tendency of the physical body to disrupt mental poise.

Pranayama (life energy control) is the fourth branch for mastery. It consists of breathing techniques resulting in controlled respiration which is characteristically deep and slow. Slow, full breathing, deliberately performed with conscious awareness, signals profound relaxation to the mind of the aspirant preparing for meditation.

Hatha Yoga

From the third and fourth stages of Patanjali's *Ashtanga Yoga* has arisen the well known and excellent school of *Hatha Yoga* with its postures and breath controls contributing to the maintenance of health or freedom from *dis-ease*.

Hatha Yoga is designed to bring into reality the dictum of 'mind over matter'. Through *Hatha Yoga* the consciousness gains rulership of its vehicle for expression, the physical body.

Pratyahara, the fifth step, is withdrawal of the senses from the stimulation of the environment as preparation for the journey into the mental space explored in meditation. It may be induced by fixing the attention upon a mental image so intensely that conscious recognition of impulses from the five sensory gates are excluded or diminished. Physical aids, such as retirement to a dark underground cave, or blocking the body orifices with cotton wool, may facilitate *Pratyahara*.

The final three stages are the jewels of yoga meditation. In these states the mind is cleared of the multitude of thoughts characteristic of normal consciousness, leaving the lake of consciousness placid.

This process is termed *Samyama* and may be likened to dropping a pebble (image concentrated upon) amongst a school of minnows (thoughts) with the result that the fish immediately flee, leaving the pebble resting on the bottom, visible through the clear, calm water of consciousness.

When the consciousness can contain a chosen mental image for approximately 12 seconds without interruption, the sixth stage of *Dharana* has been reached. This is more difficult than may appear. Subtle breaks in concentration occur, such as the thought 'I am doing this well' or 'twelve seconds must be up.'

Dhyana, the seventh phase, is sustained *Dharana* (or steadiness of concentration) for over two minutes.

Samadhi – 'with Pure Consciousness'

The last stage, *Samadhi*, may occur at any moment in a spiritual disciple's life or it may be the culmination of diligent practice of the previous seven steps. The word itself means 'with (*sam*) pure consciousness (*adhi*)'. The Sanscrit root *adhi* has been compared with the Hebrew *adoni*, meaning 'Lord' and hence *Samadhi* may be thought of as an experience of cosmic consciousness dwelling with God.

In this state, the yogin becomes one with the object meditated upon and loses awareness of separateness between the self, the object of attention, and the process of attending. *Samadhi* is the return to paradise lost.

Patanjali's *Ashtanga Yoga* had been summed up by a very clever Englishman as simply to 'Sit still, shut up, stop thinking, and go away.' Excellent advice!

The technique of meditation is not difficult but like any worth-while practice it requires perseverence, effortless effort and time. Daily meditation is a vital necessity, totally missing from our Western way of living.

Each day we waste our mental energies with negative emotion, useless day-dreaming, and gossip. Even talking about projects – or intellectualizing – drains our energy, preventing us from actually 'doing' or 'accomplishing' in life. The philosophical student should be reminded of the injunction that what comes out of the mouth is more important than what goes into it.

Interior Depths

Yoga mind control offers a state of consciousness accessible to all, in which ceaseless mental chatter is finally stilled and we plunge into the interior depths of our minds to find rejuvenation of the nervous system and a new awareness of living.

Meditation takes us upon the journey into inner space which is as limitless and infinite as outer space. The particular method used, mostly concentration upon sound or visual imagery, varies in each tradition, but whatever the technique, it may be considered as a navigational aid, bringing us to the shores of meditative experience.

Meditation is not one experience but many experiences. Bliss, creative thinking, meaningful emotional experience and heightened sensory awareness, all form some of the concrete results of meditation.

The absolute criteria for validity of psychic or

spiritual experience lies in the integrating, settling effect upon all levels of the meditator's personality. Those who experience real meditative states are loath to discuss their experiences, as opposed to those who manifest their personality disturbances, which they interpret as 'spiritual experience'.

We initiate in a particularly potent form of meditation known as *Surya Shabda* or 'listening to the solar currents'. These 'currents' are inner, subtle sounds heard in the right hemisphere of the brain and related to the flow of certain nerve channels originating in the right sympathetic ganglion, which – together with the left sympathetic ganglion – form a 'Jacob's ladder' to 'heaven' on either side of the spine.

The classical texts compare focusing upon internal sounds in the head to luring a deer (the restless mind) with a hunter's flute (*nada* or inner music) into a snare or trap to be slain (thought dies).

Sound Has No External Reality

All sound exists only in the mind and has no external reality. If a tree falls in the forest without anyone being in the vicinity, does it make a noise? *No*! The tree drops as silently as a feather, for the movement produces air vibrations only – not sound vibrations.

Until shock waves travelling through the air are picked up by the ear and changed into mechanical vibrations, which in turn are converted into electrical impulses (in the temporal love of the brain), producing what we call 'sound', nothing is heard. When we search for inner sound we force the awareness to cut through the 27 layers of mind like a knife cutting through an onion to the core.

To begin practising the most elementary aspect of the *Surya Shabda kriya* (or technique), sit comfortably in a quiet, darkened room with your elbows resting upon a table or on your knees. *Lick* the thumbs (moistening them thoroughly) and then screw them firmly into the ears, letting the fingers cover the eyes without pressing upon the eyeballs. External noise and light should now be eliminated.

Focus your attention upon your right ear and begin listening for inner sound. Do not analyse the sounds you hear but simply accept them, searching underneath each manifestation for a yet more delicate sound, thus carrying yourself deeper and deeper within the cavern of the mind-brain complex.

As with all meditative *kriya*, initial patience and quiet perseverance is necessary. Practise ten minutes the first week, increasing by five minutes each week until daily practise is half-an-hour.

Ten Billion Cells
The human brain contains some ten billion cells, of which only ten per cent (or a billion) are utilized in daily living. *Surya Shabda*, when fully initiated into, opens up the 'psychic' or dormant areas of the right cerebral cortex, raising energy levels throughout the mind-body maze and releasing fuller intellectual, emotional potential.

Personal initiation into *Surya Shabda kriya* involves the giving of a *shakti* ('power') mantra which vibrates the cerebral area, making it literally slop in neuro-secretions, soma, amrita ('juices of immortality'), instantly relieving tension, dispersing negative emotion and dropping blood-pressure.

Initiates are taught the mapping of 27 layers to the consciousness and the meaning of each type of sound heard while practising *Surya Shabda*. As the meditation experience deepens, synaesthesia (translation of one sensory modality into another), occurs – with the inner sounds becoming inner light, until ultimately *Samadhi* ensues.

Yamas and Niyamas

The doctrine of *Yama* and *Niyama* has been so crudely interpreted in popular Hinduism and in popular Western Yoga that it has been thought to be mere morals and dogmas. Such simplistic attitudes simply do not work.

When the *Yamas* and *Niyamas* are taken to be a set of rules for moral behaviour, we are faced with a very profound problem. It is not possible for man to be perfect in the moralistic sense. It is not in the nature of the animal. In every man, no matter how highly developed, are the basic uncivilized instincts deep in the intact brain, and as long as they are there the possibility exists of the crisis situation which will release them.

I have found out two things about humans by my own personal experience; in every man there exists twin buttons. One of these buttons I call the 'killer button' and the other I term the 'Judas button'.

The 'killer button' is an emotional response for a certain area of the brain and when it is found in a man (normally by pushing that button with words), you can turn the most innocuous, the most passive, the most harmless person into a killer. The 'Judas button' is related to the particular flaw in each of us, which — when it is pressed — will lead us to betray the *Christos*, the higher consciousness that is in each of us.

Subtle Inner Processes

This whole doctrine of *Yama* and *Niyama* is not a rule about moral conduct. It is a guide about subtle inner processes for controlling the ebb and flow of psychic content in the inner being. When we start analyzing them, we find they have a deeper meaning beyond the popular, external mass meaning.

If we look at the first *Yama* (control), it is *Ahimsa*, which literally means non-violence. From a simplistic view it is equated with the Commandment 'Thou shalt not kill'. Yet within each one of us a button can be pressed in some crisis situation in life when we become capable of killing – Yoga or no Yoga.

One of the basic Buddhist injunctions is a form of *Ahimsa:* 'Thou shalt kill no living thing.' Yet if you take quinine to cure malaria, you kill certain parasites floating around in your bloodstream. If you are a Jain (who rings a little bell to scare away the insects as he treads on the grass), are you breaking your vows on non-violence if you use penicillin to overcome the micro-organisms causing an attack of pneumonia? If a man is in a position in life where he must kill, where he feels that to kill is righteous or justifiable, is he breaking the rule of *Ahimsa?* Does *Ahimsa* mean literally – no physical killing?

Given a little thought, it is obvious that the whole thing is a joke if it does not mean a little more than that. What is it in man that is not to be killed? What non-violence means, what *Ahimsa* means, is an attitude of mind – not a set of actions. It is the attitude in the mind, not the action, that determines the *Karma.*

And what is it that each man is prone to kill? It is his higher consciousness. What is the killer of the higher consciousness? It is the negative emotions. He who esoterically practises *Ahimsa* tries not to permit violence against the higher consciousness or to kill it by the misuse and abuse of the emotional faculties.

Satya – Truth

The second *Yama* is *Satya* – Truth. It is a familiar moral injunction to always tell the truth – at an external level. Now man is possessed of a very curious thing. It is called the unconscious mind. As each of us reads this, we are operating with approximately one-tenth of our total mental activity,because – like an iceberg – nine-tenths of our mind is submerged. What man can claim to know the contents of that submerged part of his mind? How do you tell when you are being truthful?

If *Satya* means non-lying, then are you practising *Satya* when you refuse to tell the white lie that saves someone from hurt? It is obvious that a simple interpretation of what constitutes the truth is not *Satya*. For that inner spiritual truth has to do with the most difficult thing that any of us can come to. And that is the truth to the Self, acknowledging the flaws, looking within and seeing what is there, facing it without fear, and going within, even if it tears a man apart.

In the West we have a particular type of Yoga that does this very successfully – yes, this is Yoga – it is called psychotherapy and it is one of the most valuable heritages that Western civilization has produced. In fact I do not believe that for Western people who are serious about Yoga there can be any Yoga in their life without – at some time – psychotherapy. That going within and facing the truth about the self and the acceptance of the self, this is *Satya*.

Asteya – Non-stealing

The third *Yama*, *Asteya*, literally means non-stealing. At a general level we say that stealing is taking that which one has not earned. I accept that each of us must earn what we possess, that if we take something that we have not earned then we are breaking *Asteya*, or the rule of non-stealing.

However, *Asteya* goes much deeper than that. Each man in his life, in his personal existence, is a vital cog in the wheel of life. Each person fulfils a potential. Each person in being part of that cog of this whole thing that we call life, fulfils *Dharma*, or obligation to life. Esoterically, he who steals, he who breaks the law of *Asteya* or non-stealing, is he who steals the time of the spirit, the time of the higher consciousness, that is meant to be devoted to the unfoldment of the higher being.

That stealing that takes place in our life is the stealing of time. From birth to death, from womb to tomb and each moment of life that we fail to struggle with ourselves, we are stealing the time of the spirit, that time of *Dharma* that has been given to us. This is the true essence of that rule of *Asteya*. Killing time isn't murder – it's spiritual suicide!

Brahmacharya – Divine Action

Fourthly there is the *Yama* of *Brahmacharya*. Perhaps of all the *Yamas* that have been written about in popular Hindu books, this has been the most misunderstood and yet it deals with the most potent essence of man's being. Fools have said that *Brahmacharya* is celibacy, that it has something to do with the banking up of sexual forces. Yet he who has any knowledge of Indian philosophy, who examines Buddhist and Tantric tradition, knows that there are other traditions in Indian philosophy besides the simplistic *Bhakti Vedantist* tradition, that belie the whole concept of *Brahmacharya* as celibacy.

In the Upanishads it is clearly indicated that the sexual potential lying within each human is communion, a divine force. The Upanishads say that the vulva is an altar and that the hairs upon the vulva are the flames upon the altar. The body is a temple and the sexual act is an act of divine worship.

And yet fools have said that *Brahmacharya* means celibacy. Consequently, whole hordes of people in India and the West are knotting themselves up sexually trying to follow this rule, thinking it means celibacy. Well, it doesn't mean that. What does it mean?

Brahma means God, *Charya* means action. And

the word itself means God-action or Divine action.
What it says is that the celibacy of sex is not in the
act, but in the attitude that is held in consciousness.
Brahmacharya is an attitude of divine worship. It has
nothing to do with the physical action itself. In the
scriptures the body is spoken of as the castle of
Brahma and in this castle we worship an inner
instinct as an aspect of the Divine self.

Freud's Discovery
Freud discovered for the Western world what the
Tantrist of India, the early Dravidians, and certain
schools of Buddhism had known for thousands of
years. He found that the primal force of power
within each of us is the sexual mainspring, that the
foundation of being lies in sexual forces. People
have badly misunderstood Freud when they
interpreted him to mean that everything has to do
with sex.

What Freud said was not that the sexual energies
were the most important thing in life, but that they
provided the power for the basis of behaviour.

Just as the wiring in a factory provides the power
for the making of its products, and if that wiring is
faulty nothing will be properly made, so if the
sexual energies that run in us through the nervous
system are faulty or twisted up, then the rest of the
activity of the human is going to be interfered with.

This is what the whole concept of *Brahmacharya* is
about. It means something very special. What it
means in each person's life I cannot tell you. At a
theoretical level it means that this worship of the
body should be for everyone, it means, if you wish,
free love. But at a personal level, in practice, this is
something that each person has to struggle to work
out for himself.

In theory we say that this divine act of expression
of love should be free, provided that no hurt accrues
and provided no uncared-for children result. That

is simple common sense. But at a deep personal
level each one has to work out the inner significance
of this for himself.

Aparigraha – Non-possession

Finally we come to the last *Yama* – *Aparigraha*,
which means non-possession. In the classical
Vedantist tradition it should mean that when a man
becomes a *Sannyasin* he abandons all wordly goods.
Now what is important about this idea of
Aparigraha? It is obvious that if you are a Westerner
living in a materialistic, commercial world, that you
cannot survive without goods. What is meant by
non-possession?

Only fools take the *Yamas* and *Niyamas* literally. It
has nothing to do with the acquisition of goods.
What it has to do with is the attitude or the
attachment to these goods. All things, all material
goods, are here for our use or for our misuse. All
goods, all fruits of the earth, all fruits of man's brain
in the sense of manufacture of material goods, are
here for enjoyment and pleasure, provided our
consciousness does not centre around acquisition.
Again, *Aparigraha* is not an act, it is an attitude of
mind. It is not a question of possessing goods –
rather, do the goods possess us?

Saucha – Purity

Now we move to the *Niyamas*. They represent the
positive element, in the sense of things to be done,
acts to be worked at, concrete realities. The first of
these is *Saucha*, which means purity. Fools have
thought that it means purity of mind. Who can say
that he has purity of mind? Only an infant, and
even then that can be argued from a certain psycho-
analytic viewpoint – only an infant has the
possibility of a pure mind, if it means the mind.

Only *Saucha* does not mean the mind. It refers to
the body. It means purity of the body in a

physiological sense. For that purity of the body, which is the vehicle for the expression of consciousness, is the removal of toxic wastes, the malas, the phlegms, that alter the nervous system of man, that clog up the consciousness, the brain. The maintenance of that purity of the body temple has to do with the ways that each one of us starts to die. There are four ways in which each man begins to die. I will talk about three of them now and the fourth one later.

Psychosomatic Diseases

The first way in which each of us begins to die physically and mentally we can call the psychosomatic act. Each of us begins to kill himself by misuse of the mind/body relationship. How? By misunderstanding and abuse of the *Yamas*, by committing those mental acts of violence, of killing our higher consciousness, by refusing to acknowledge the truth of the self, by stealing the time that has been given to us from birth to death, by misusing the nervous system in its sexual function, by becoming attracted to physical goods and suffering the tension of their loss.

Perhaps 60 to 70 per cent of people who come to doctors are suffering from psychosomatic diseases, a disease process that started from emotion tensions.

The second way we start to die has to do with the fundamental care of our being, the nucleus of the cell. It is currently thought in Western biology that individual cell death is programmed in the chromosomes. We suspect that the practices of Yoga may be able to alter the programming in the very nucleus of the cell and thus prolong the physical act of life.

The third way that we start to die has particularly to do with *Saucha* or purity. It is simply this: we begin to die at a cellular level by drowning in our own excreta. The semi-permeable membrane of the cell wall becomes clogged with wastes and loses its ability to take in nutrients and throw out waste products.

The practices of *Hatha Yoga*, the internal cleansings, the internal massage of the postures, diet and fasting, maintain the health of the cell wall and prevent its deterioration. *Saucha*-purity means consistent removal of internal wastes from the physical body, to prolong life and cleanse the nervous system for higher states.

Santosha – Contentment

The second *Niyama*, *Santosha*, means contentment – the practice of being contented. How? By living in present time, forgetting the past, leaving the daydreams of the future, keeping the energies of the mind/body complex for the present moment. We can cultivate contentment by using the twilight period between waking and sleep and between sleep and full waking, to seed our unconscious mind with positive suggestions of happiness. What is this thing called Yoga?

The oldest definition of Yoga is the cessation of the fluctuations of the mind, those wanderings, those tensions, those emotional jumps. He who practises Yoga is he who can pull the mind together to stop those fluctuations. He who can reach inside himself to bring out the energies, regardless of what has happened, he who can have the hounds of hell chase him in his mind and tear him to pieces and can stop these fluctuations of that mind when necessary, has Yoga.

Tapas – Indifference

The third of the *Niyamas* is called *Tapas*, roughly translated as indiference. *Tapas* is the practice of indifference to discomfort when no useful purpose is served by taking notice of that discomfort. For instance, a simple and useful way to begin the practice of *Tapas* is to start taking cold showers to stimulate the nervous system.

Swadhyaya – Self study

The fourth *Niyama* is *Swadhyaya* – self study. Its inner essence deals with the fourth way we begin to die. This self-study means that the act of living is a continuous process of learning. Stop learning and you begin to die in a very special way. Psychologists know that at least 50 per cent of senility is psychological, loss of interest in life, loss of willingness to learn by life's experience. In this context Yoga is a form of re-education.

The Final Process

The final process of *Ishwarapranidhana* – crudely interpreted – means devotion to God. In *Samkhyan* terms it means devotion to the Self as the essence of God. For what is God? It is that on-going life process. It is no being, no person, it is this whole process of life and life awareness. And he who practises *Ishwarapranidhana* is devoted to the on-going process of life and evolution in himself.

For Yoga to survive in an intelligent way for thoughtful people in the West, a new recasting must come about. The classical texts of Yoga are the testimonies of Indian civilization at its greatest peak. India is a badly decayed civilization at the moment, but it has left us a heritage in the classical scriptures which are short, succinct statements for the minds of future ages to expand, expound and enlarge upon.

Some schools have made morals and dogmas out of the classical scriptures. Let them. Those who want simplistic Yoga, let them have it. But those who want to find out what it is really about are involved in becoming builders and recasters of this thing called Yoga.

SANSKRIT GLOSSARY

A

Ahimsa: 'Non-killing'. The Indian doctrine of non-violence and non-injury. The first *Yama* (control) of the first stage of *Ashtanga Yoga*.

Ajna: 'Non-knowledge'. The sixth psychic centre physically indicated by the pituitary gland and the cavernous plexus. Some authors have associated the pineal gland with *Ajna*, but the clue to the correct correlation is given in the symbol of *Ajna* as a two-petalled lotus – the two petals corresponding to the anterior and posterior pituitary lobes.

Akasa: The fifth element ether symbolized by a black oval. The *tattwa* of *Vishuddha chakra*.

Anahata: 'Non-sound' or 'Unstruck sound'. The fourth psychic centre indicated physically by the thymus gland and the cardiac plexus.

Antar-Anga: 'Inner limbs'. The four higher phases of *Ashtanga Yoga* comprising *Pratyahara, Dharana, Dhyana* and *Samadhi*.

Apas: The second element water symbolized by a silver crescent. The *tattwa* of *Swadhisthana*.

Asana: 'Seat'. The group of eighty-four classical body postures or exercises taught in *Hatha Yoga*.

Ashtanga Yoga: 'Eight-limbed' Yoga. A term applied to the system outlined in Patanjali's *Yoga Sutras* wherein Yoga is divided into eight steps or stages: *Yama* (control), *Niyama* (Moral observances), *Asana* (posture), *Pranayama* (breath control), *Pratyahara* (sense withdrawal), *Dharana* (concentration), *Dhyana* (sustained concentration), and *Samadhi* (mental union or equilibrium).

Audgita: The silent or mental chanting of a mantra.

B

Bahira-Anga: 'Outer limbs'. The four lower phases of *Ashtanga Yoga* comprising *Yama, Niyama, Asana* and *Pranayama*.

Bhakti: That path of Yoga which seeks realization through the practice of devotion and love in both a religious (*Bhakti*) and a philosophical (*Parabhakti*) sense.

Bija: 'Seed'. The root sound of each *chakra* which, when intoned as a mantra, will release its psychic energy. The *Bija* mantras of the first five *chakras* are Lang, Vang (chanted 'Wang'), Rang, Yang, and Hang.

Bramacharya: In Yoga the fourth *Yama* or discipline of the first stage (*Yama*) of *Ashtanga Yoga*. Generally understood as the observance of strict sexual celibacy but is better interpreted as moderation and control of passion.

C

Chakra: 'Wheel, disc, whirlpool'. The term is applied to the basic seven psychic centres outlined in Yoga and Tantra. *Chakra* implies a vortex and thus we may define a psychic centre as a 'whirling vortex of psychic energy at the conjunction points of the mind and the body.'

D

Dharana: 'Concentration'. The sixth stage of *Ashtanga Yoga*.

Dhyana: 'Sustained concentration'. The seventh stage of *Ashtanga Yoga* and an advanced state of *Dharana*. Some have applied the English words 'contemplation' and 'meditation' to *Dhyana*, but the classical Yoga texts state that so many *Dharanas* (measured in a specific time unit) equal one *Dhyana* and in turn so many *Dhyanas* equal one *Samadhi*.

The essential difference between *Dharana* and *Dhyana* is of degree rather than kind.

G

Gnana: That path of Yoga which seeks realization through the pursuit of philosophical knowledge.

H

Ham Sa: A mantra affirming 'I am He' or 'I am Brahman'. This mantra is one of the most potent methods of releasing positive emotional attitudes from the subconscious.

I

Ida' One of the three major psychic nerves or *nadis*. *Ida* runs up the left side of the spinal column and is the channel of negative emotional energy.

J

Japa: The practice of driving mantric affirmations deep into the subconscious through constant repetition, either silently or audibly.

K

Karma Yoga: The path of Yoga seeking realization through detachment from the fruits of all action and dedicating all activity to *Ishvara* (anthropomorphic aspect of God). *Karma* as a doctrine, is the recognition of the fundamental laws of action and reaction in human affairs.

Kundalini: Latent nerve energy within the central nervous system. Symbolically and allegorically represented by a snake coiled three-and-a-half times.

L

Laya Yoga: 'Rhythm, absorption'. That branch of Yoga dealing with the arousal, release and control of latent nerve energy (*kundalini*) hidden (absorbed) within man's nervous system.

M

Manipura‘ 'Gem city'. The third psychic centre physically represented by the pancreas and the solar plexus.

Mantra Yoga: The systematic use of sound vibration to bring about physical and mental changes.

Marmasthanani: The sixteen vital body areas that are concentrated upon in certain exercises of *Raja* and *Hatha Yoga*.

Mritasana: 'Dead pose'. Another name for the relaxation posture popularly known as *Savasana*.

Muladhara: 'Root base'. The first psychic centre physically represented by the testes or ovaries and the sacral plexus.

N

Nadi: 'Motion'. A psychic or astral nerve tube. Yoga teaches that seventy-two thousand such *nadis* exist in the psychic counterpart of the gross body.

Nadisuddhi: The purification of the *nadis* through conjoined breathing and mental exercises.

P

Padma: 'Lotus'. Another term for the psychic centres. *Padma* refers to the potential growth and development of our psychic centres, just as a lotus bulb is capable of development into a lotus in full bloom.

Padmasana: 'Lotus pose'. An advanced footlock suitable for meditation. The symmetrical arrangement of the legs produced by placing the right foot on the left thigh and the left foot on the right thigh is said to resemble a lotus flower.

Parang Mukhi: 'Turning away'. Another term for *Yoni Mudra*.

Patanjali: The author of *Yoga Sutras* who lived in the second century B.C. He is responsible for the division of Yoga into eight distinct branches or stages and as a result his outline of Yoga is known as *Ashtanga*.

Pingala: One of the three major *nadis*. *Pingala* runs up the right side of the spinal column and is the channel of positive emotional energy.

Prana: 'Breath, life, wind, energy, spirit, power.'

Pranayama: The control of life force (*prana*) through the regulation of the respiratory process.

Prithivi: The first element earth, symbolized by a yellow square. The *tattwa* of *Muladhara*.

R

Raja Yoga: 'Kingly or Royal Yoga.' The science of creating a mergence or union (Yoga) between the conscious and subconscious mind, thus producing a third state which becomes 'Superconsciousness'.

S

Saguna: 'With form'. Concentration upon a definite form or something of a very concrete nature.

Sahasrara: 'Thousand-petalled'. The seventh psychic centre physically indicated by the pineal gland and the cerebrum (containing thousands of cells or 'petals'). *Sahasrara* is said to be the dwelling-place of *Shiva*, the destroyer of ignorance (*Maya*). This is an esoteric statement concerning the ability of man to destroy ignorance (*Maya*) by the use of his enlightened consciousness (*Shiva*) which results from the awakening of *Sahasrara chakra*.

Samadhi: 'With God'. The state of consciousness resulting from the contact of the individual consciousness with Universal consciousness. In terms of Jung's psychology, *Samadhi* would be the emergence of the 'Collective Unconsciousness'. *Samadhi* is the final stage of *Ashtanga Yoga* and the goal of all Yoga.

Samyama: The three higher phases of *Ashtanga Yoga*. These are *Dharana, Dhyana,* and *Samadhi*.

San Mukhi: 'Six orifices'. Another term for *Yoni Mudra*.

Savasana: 'Corpse pose'. The technique of consciously relaxing the body, section by section. An exercise of immense value for neurasthenia, exhaustion, insomnia, hypertension, and high blood-pressure. It is particularly efficacious if combined with certain mental exercises.

Shakti: Divine energy in its manifested form and considered as feminine. Christians speak of the 'Fatherhood of God' and Hindus speak of the 'Motherhood of God'. The bridge between these two concepts is the bridge between materialism and spirituality.

Shushumna: The major *nadi* corresponding to the spinal cord. The channel of 'Christ consciousness' through which *kundalini* ascends to unite with *Sahasrara*.

Siddhis: The psychic powers that develop as the student advances along the path of Yoga. Undeveloped abilities which most people are unaware of possessing.

Sukhasana: 'Easy pose'. Simple cross-legged position for meditation and neuromuscular training.

Swadhisthana: 'One's own place'. The second psychic centre physically indicated by the adrenal glands and hypogastric plexus.

T

Tantra: 'System, ritual, doctrine, loom'. The original philosophy of the Dravidian inhabitants of India. Now considered the revealed teaching for this age (*Kali Yoga*), *Tantra* contains the deepest doctrines and the most potent techniques of Indian philosophy.

Tattwa: 'Quality'. The essence or quality of any given substance.

Tejas: The third element, Fire, symbolized by a

red triangle with the apex down. The *tattwa* of *Manipura*.

U

Udgita: Verbal intonation of a mantra.

V

Vayu: The fourth element, air, symbolized by a blue hexagon. The *tattwa* of *Anahata*.

Vishuddha: 'Purity centre'. The fifth psychic centre physically represented by the thyroid gland and the cervical plexus.

Y

Yantra: A geometrical design used for concentration, ritual or as an amulet. A mandala tends to be circular and always contains the figure of a deity or animal as distinct from the purely abstract lines and curves of the yantra.

Yoga: 'Union'. The science of mental, physical and universal integration. From the Sanskrit root of yoga we derive the English 'yoke', which not only implies a linking with cosmic forces but also suggests the harnessing (a yoke is a harness) and control of man's own energies.

Yoga-Nidra: A deep state of dreamless sleep attained by certain mental exercises peculiar to Yoga.

Yoni Mudra: 'Womb symbol'. One of the most important keys to Yoga psychosomatic practices.